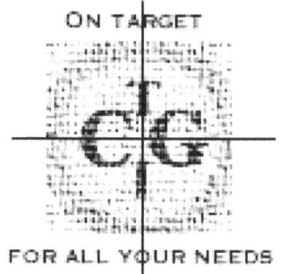

ON TARGET

FOR ALL YOUR NEEDS

# THE CANCER GROUP INSTITUTE

23825 Anza Avenue
Suite. #108
Torrence, California – 90505
© 2017

**www.CancerGroup.com**

# BREAST CANCER

## Disclaimer

*CancerGroup.com* serves only as a clearinghouse for medical and health information and does not directly or indirectly practice medicine. Any information provided by *CancerGroup.com* is intended solely for educating our clients and should not be construed as medical advice or guidance, which should always be obtained from a physician or other licensed health care professional. As such, the client assumes full responsibility for the appropriate use of medical information contained in this book and agrees to hold *CancerGroup.com* and any of its third party providers harmless from any and all claims or actions arising from clients' use or reliance on this guide. Although *CancerGroup.com* makes every reasonable attempt to conduct a thorough search of the published medical literature, the possibility exists that some significant articles may be missed. The statements found throughout have not been evaluated by the Food and Drug Administration. These products are not intended to diagnose, treat, cure, or prevent any disease.

Any uncontrolled growth of breast tissue cells, which has the capacity to spread, **is** breast cancer. Early breast cancer is confined to the breast and

the tumor is not larger than 5 cm (about 2 inches) across.

It may also involve the lymph glands under the armpit, called the **axillary lymph nodes**.

Sidebar. I have known women who shave their underarms with a wet razor, and in doing so the new hair follicle **might** grow **back** into the skin causing a **small lump** to present (appear).

**This is nothing to worry about.** However if it doesn't disappear by your next monthly check, then a visit to your Dr. is recommended, just for your peace of mind.

Any disease, problem or trouble that G-d gives has a cure. It is basically up to us to find the right person/physician who can channel these cures.

The cure is always available; we just have to know where to look.

In its most simplistic terms, any math question has a correct answer, its' up to us to find it. We may not understand the mathematics behind the problem, but its answer is available.

This formula, which I name the "**Braham Theory of Discovery**", is correct across every dimension and disease known and even not known to man.

This is how the "**Braham Theory of Discovery**" works in action.

The cure is always available; we just have to know where to look.

It has not spread to any distant sites in the body, as far as can be told with today's technology. **Locally Advanced Breast Cancer** is noted by a tumor greater than 5 cm across, or a fixed lump in the axilla representing cancer, ulceration of the skin from cancer, or involvement of the deep chest muscles.

**Inflammatory Breast Cancer** is a hot, tender breast with skin looking like an orange peel, called peau de orange and almost always has spread to the axilla.

**Metastatic breast cancer** means the disease **has spread** to other areas of the body, such as the lung, liver, brain, skin or bone.

Breast cancer, like other cancers, **starts in just a single cell**. Normally, breast cells divide infrequently after breast growth is completed; only to replace those cells lost through old age or injury.

The production of new breast cells from pre-existing ones is under tight control by the genetic code, or genes, of each cell. When this code becomes damaged, a cell may start dividing out of control. The breast cancer cell is genetically damaged, but otherwise it looks very similar to normal body tissue.

This is why our immune system may fail to detect it as abnormal. These cells can pile up to form a local tumor. A tumor simply means a swelling; it is not necessarily cancerous. Less than 1/3 of new breast lumps and bumps are cancer.

A **tumor** which only grows in its place or origin, and cannot spread distantly, is called **benign** and **is not cancer**. However, a tumor which has the capacity to spread (whether it actually does or not) is called **malignant**, this is cancer.

The actual process of spread is called metastasis. It is this ability to spread to any organ in the body which makes cancers so dangerous.

**How Common is Breast Cancer?**

Breast cancer is the most common cancer in women, after skin cancer, the median age at diagnosis for cancer of the breast is 61 years of age. The median age at death for cancer of the breast is 68 years of age.

Approximately 252,710 new cases of invasive breast cancer will be diagnosed in women, while about 63,410 new cases of carcinoma in situ (CIS) will be diagnosed (CIS is non-invasive and is the **earliest form of breast cancer**).

Approximately 40,170 women will die from breast cancer, which makes it the second leading cause of cancer death after lung cancer in women.

About 2,470 new cases of invasive breast cancer are expected to be diagnosed in men in 2017. A man's lifetime risk of breast cancer is about 1 in 1,000.

The number of annual deaths from breast cancer has remained about the same for the past 50 years, although the number of cases is increasing.

However, there is some **decrease** due to less use of hormone replacement therapy (HRT) after the results of the Women's Health Initiative were published in 2002. This study linked HRT use to an increased risk of breast cancer and heart diseases.

This shows the benefits of early detection, which impacts survival. Also, effective treatment is increasing survival in all breast cancer patients. One in nine women will get breast cancer in the U.S.A. during their lifetimes.

Two thirds to 75% of cases are Early Breast Cancer, 20% are Advanced Breast Cancer (including Metastatic), and 5% are the Inflammatory subtype.

Initial Early Breast Cancer which was thought cured may be detected as the Advanced Metastatic type decades after the initial diagnosis and treatment. Advanced Breast cancer can smolder along, slowly growing in the bone, for many years before detection.

## What Causes or Increases the Risk for Breast Cancer?

Like any other cancer, the exact reason why one woman gets breast cancer and another doesn't remains unknown. However, **certain risk factors** have been identified:

**1)** Being female (only 1% of cases are in males).
**2)** Family history of breast cancer in mother and aunts; BRCA-1 gene. The BRCA-1 gene stands for breast cancer, and although the risk is increased with the gene, not all patients with it get breast cancer. Also, genes for rare diseases like ataxia-telangectasia (A-T) (lack of repair of skin to sun damage) associated with breast CA.
**3)** Getting older-- average age is 60 to get breast cancer.
**4)** Lots of estrogens-- including start of menstrual periods at a young age completion of menstrual periods at an old age, no children or first child after age 30, being obese (fat cells produce estrogen).
**5)** Low dose radiation exposure-- can take 10 to 50 years afterward to develop breast cancer, among others. About 6 per 1 million women are estimated to get breast cancer from the mammogram radiation, but this is believed worthwhile owing to the many early cancers found.

**6)** High fat in the diet. This many also be related to obesity above.
**7)** Tobacco smoking, alcohol or birth control pills do NOT seem to increase risk!

### Is Breast Cancer Preventable?

Despite advances in the diagnosis and treatment of breast cancer, one third of the women who develop breast cancer will die of the disease.

Recognition of this limitation of currently available therapies has resulted in a new focus on breast cancer prevention. At present, the only method of prevention that is available in routine clinical practice is prophylactic mastectomy.

However, little agreement exists on the efficacy of this procedure or the appropriate indications for its use. Both subcutaneous and simple (**total**) **mastectomy,** have been employed for **prophylaxis** (A measure taken for the prevention of a disease or condition.)

In a subcutaneous mastectomy, the breast parenchyma is removed through an incision in the inframammary crease, preserving the nipple-areolar complex. With this approach, breast tissue must be left behind under the nipple and areola to prevent their **devascularization**, which is the interruption of circulation of blood to a part due to obstruction of blood vessels, and access to the periphery of the breast (axillary tail, subclavicular area) is often very difficult.

One study of 12 subcutaneous mastectomies done on cadavers demonstrated retained breast tissue in 83% of cases. There are multiple reports of breast cancer occurring in women following subcutaneous mastectomy.

Laboratory studies support the clinical concern that a reduction in the volume of breast tissue may not be associated with a proportionate reduction in breast cancer risk.

The alternative to subcutaneous mastectomy **is total or simple mastectomy**, in which an ellipse of skin including the nipple-areola complex is removed to allow removal of the breast tissue.

Although it is likely that **100% of the breast tissue** is **NOT** removed with this procedure, removal of the nipple-areola complex clearly decreases the amount of residual breast tissue.

When prophylactic simple mastectomy is undertaken, meticulous attention to the removal of all possible breast tissue is very important.

The procedure should be similar to a therapeutic mastectomy and should **include** the use of thin skin flaps. You should mention this to your Physician **BEFORE** surgery commences.

Unfortunately, there are no large clinical studies of the risk of breast cancer **after** prophylactic simple mastectomy.

The many drawbacks to the wide spread use of **prophylactic mastectomy** as a **prevention** strategy are apparent.

Researchers have focused their attention into the development and testing of **chemopreventive agents\***, which I will speak about later in this publication.

\*The use of a drug or compound to interfere with a disease process, for example, cancer **chemopreventive agents** — agents used to inhibit, delay, or reverse carcinogenesis.

Patient selection for **breast-conserving treatment** involves an assessment of whether the primary tumor can be **successfully** removed with an acceptable cosmetic result.

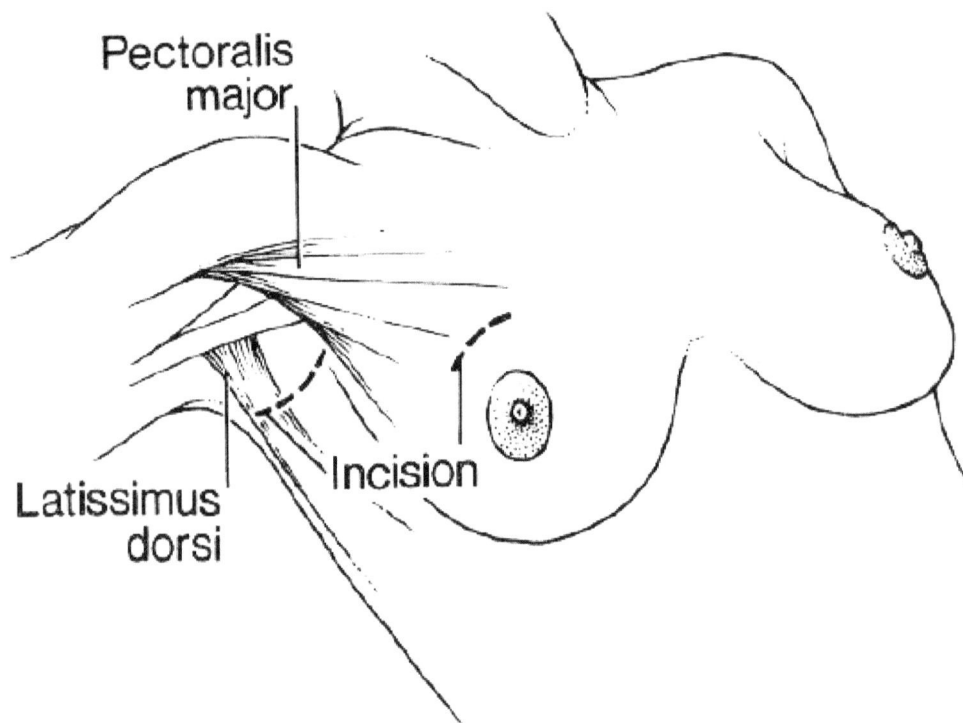

This shows Breast conserving surgery with axillary dissection

Along with the estimate of the risk of local recurrence following breast-conserving treatment and mastectomy, and **very importantly**, an evaluation of the patient's desires and expectations.

Evaluation of these factors requires a complete medical history, not just your history, but also your family's medical history in order to complete a true picture.

Also a complete physical examination, along with a detailed mammographic evaluation (ideally with magnification views and prior to surgical biopsy) to exclude the presence of other lesions in the breast and to help define the extent of the primary tumor, and careful pathologic evaluation of the resected breast specimen.

Most of the risk factors for getting Breast Cancer are not in a woman's control. In the past, women with a very high risk sometimes had both breasts removed as a preventative measure, called **prophylactic mastectomy**.

This is very infrequent today, given the earlier detection and better treatment of breast cancer. Reducing fat in the diet, getting pregnant in her early 20's, and appropriate screening and prompt treatment can reduce cancer deaths.

**How Does My Doctor Screen For Breast Cancer?**
There are two common ways of screening for breast cancer. Every woman must do a **Breast Self Exam** one week **after** her menstrual period **each month**, feeling for **lumps**.

**How to do a proper exam monthly is to first:**

1. Stand in front of a mirror with breasts exposed.
2. Raise arms above your head. Look for dimpling, swelling, soreness, or redness in all parts of your breasts in the mirror.

3. Repeat with hands placed on hips.

4. Palpate your breasts with your fingers, feeling for lumps. Try

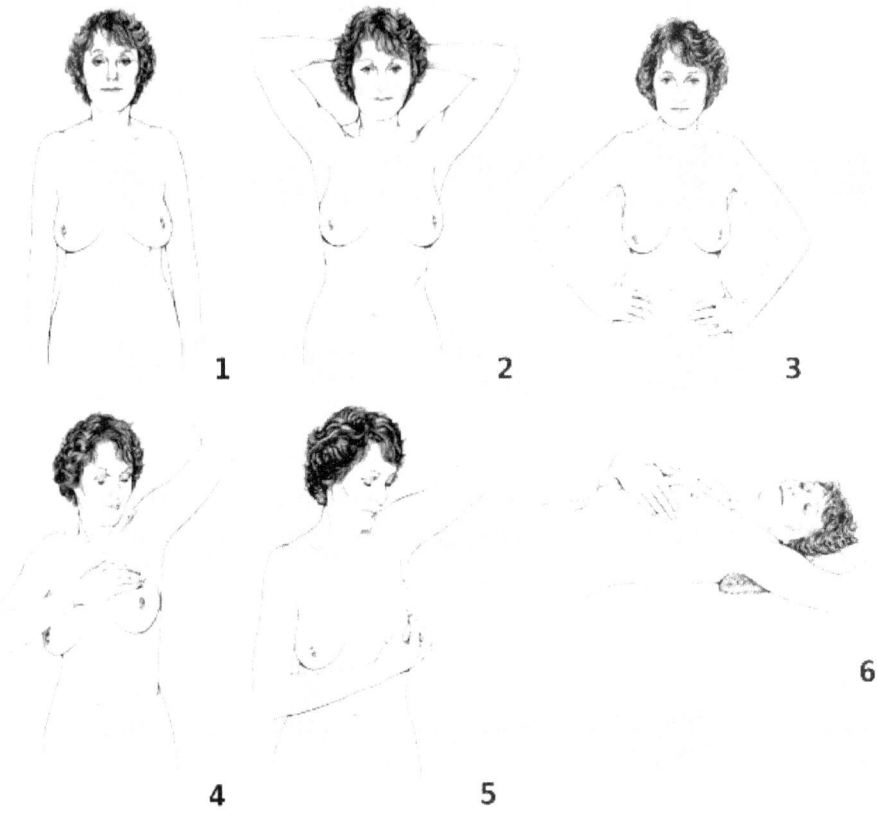

**After menopause**, it can be done at any standard time each month. This should also be done if a patient with a history of breast cancer has kept a breast. The American Cancer Society recommends a baseline mammogram at age 35-40 with one done every other year from ages 40 to 50.

A Picture tell a thousand words, so below are more examples of breast self exam, and what to look for if your breasts are producing a discharge.

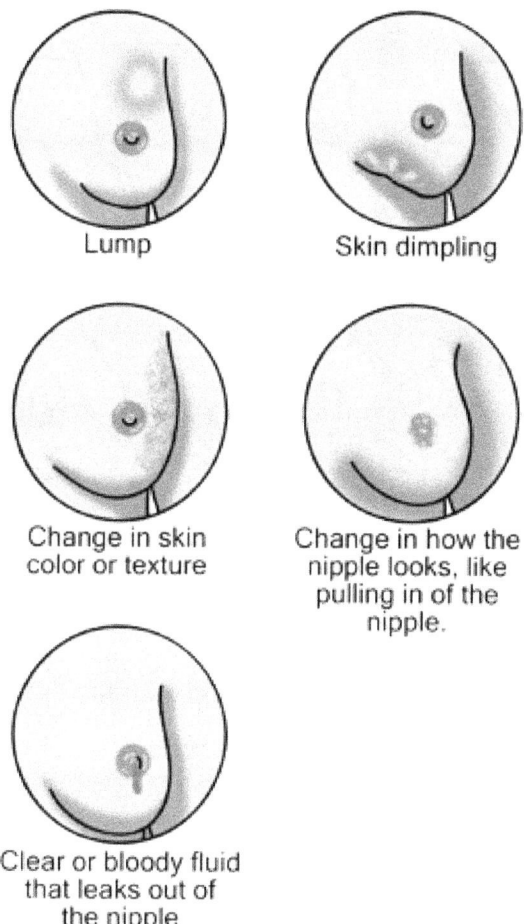

Lump

Skin dimpling

Change in skin color or texture

Change in how the nipple looks, like pulling in of the nipple.

Clear or bloody fluid that leaks out of the nipple

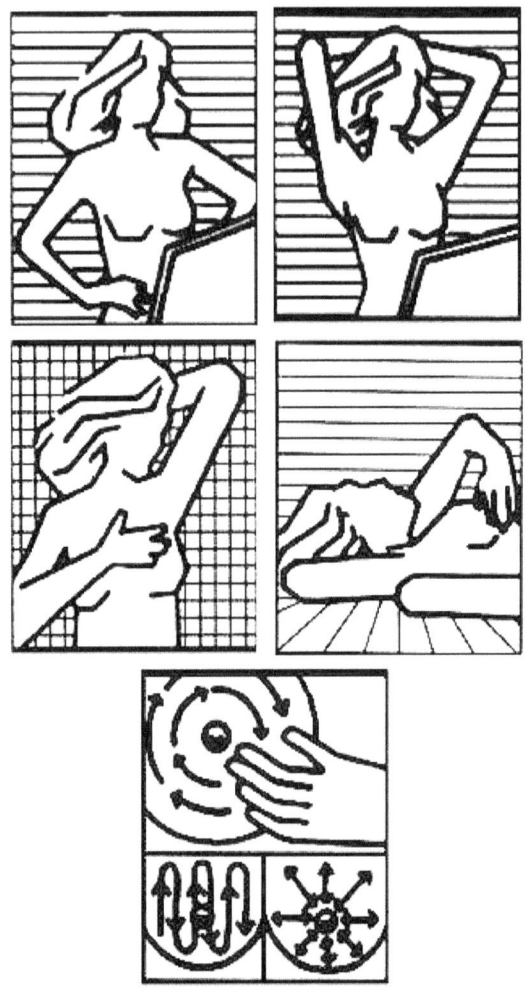

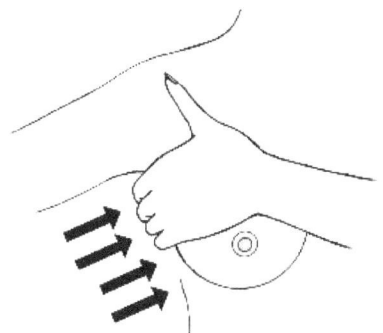

Pump directly into armpit.
Feel for tenderness.
Repeat pumping action 10X - 20X

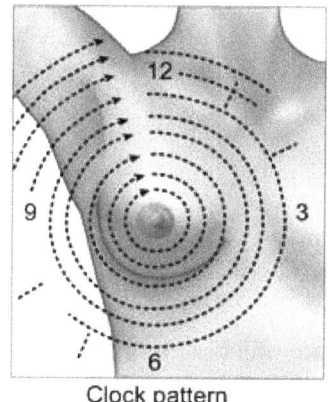

Clock pattern

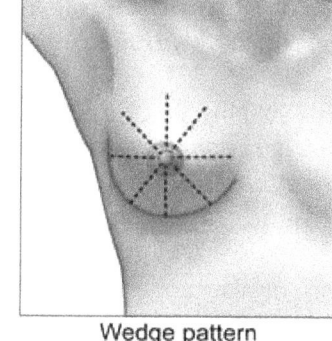

Wedge pattern

Women aged greater than >50, should get a mammogram every year. Women at higher risk may get this test more frequently, as should women who have **had** breast cancer but kept their breast.

In spite of the recent controversy for how often to get mammograms, the main point is to get them on a regular basis, especially as a woman gets older than age 40.

One very important strategy in reducing the risk for breast cancer is the use of screening to achieve earlier detection of breast cancer.

**Earlier diagnosis** is thought by many Physicians to be the motivating factor to obtain treatment **before** metastasis occurs, and thus thereby avert death due to the disease.

**What are the Symptoms of Breast Cancer?**

**Early breast cancer usually has no symptoms**, but is picked up with screening tests. It is important to note that most new breast lumps are not cancer, but it must be ruled out anyway.

The **first symptom** is usually a new lump or bump in the breast, which is of dominant character. This means that it is **single, hard, non-movable, non-tender**, and in only **one breast**.

Occasionally (5%) breast cancer results in a nipple discharge, while 50% of watery discharges are from cancer, only 1% of milky or pussy discharges are cancerous. In more advanced breast cancer, the breast may have a large tumor, or have a lump in the armpit.

Inflammatory breast cancer looks like an infection, being red and painful, and may be confused with the much more common mastitis, which is a simple breast infection. Breast cancer spread to bones can cause pain and fractures, and to the brain can result in symptoms of imbalance, confusion, headache and local weakness or numbness.

Rarely, it spreads to the eyes to cause blindness. Most commonly, however, it stays localized in the breast for many years. If it spreads, it is most commonly to bone where it may remain unapparent for many years. About 5% of patients develop cancers in both breasts, called bilateral breast cancer.

## How Does Breast Cancer Spread?

It generally starts inside the milk ducts of the breast, then it invades through the wall of the breast. If it invades, then it grows locally to form a tumor, and the first spread is to the lymph glands in same sided armpit (called the axilla).

When the tumor is 1 inch across, there is a 30% chance that it has spread to the axillary lymph glands; when it is 2 inches across, the chance of the axilla being involved, or positive is about 60%.

Once the axilla is involved, the cancer is considered **systemic,** that is likely to have spread to other areas of the body through the bloodstream. The most common places for it to spread, in order, are the bones, liver, lung, skin and brain.

## What are the Types of Breast Cancer?

The most common type is called **Invasive Ductal Carcinoma**, that is, the cancer starts in the milk duct and invades through it. This accounts for 80% of breast cancers, and is the only type **found in men.**

It accounts for most of the locally advanced and inflammatory cancer too. The next most common type is called **Invasive Lobular Carcinoma,** it arises from the lobules in the breast and accounts for 10% of cases.

Alternatively, the either the Ductal or the Lobular type of cancers may not invade, but stay locally within the ducts or lobules and grow to a large size there.

Non-invasive or in Situ disease accounts for about 14% of breast cancer, it **does not spread** to the axilla or elsewhere, and in general patients do better than with invasive disease. It is also important because local recurrence of breast cancer (after breast conservation therapy) may be of this non-invasive type and so less dangerous.

**Ductal Carcinoma in Situ**, or DCIS for short, is becoming more common since it often can only be detected with a mammogram.

Interestingly, Lobular Carcinoma in Situ, or LCIS for short, is a marker for the development of later invasive ductal cancer, which happens in 30% of patients.

**Uncommon types** of breast cancer include medullary, mucinous and tubular forms, which all tend to occur in older women and are less aggressive, and **Paget's Disease** of the Nipple, which appears as a scaly irritation but has an underlying lump in the breast 76% of the time.

Rarely, cancer may arise from the sweat glands of the breast (apocrine) from the immune cells in the breast (lymphoma) or from the muscle (sarcoma).

The treatment for these cancers is different than the typical ductal or lobular types. There may be a mixture of types about 16% of cases.

**How is Breast Cancer Detected and Evaluated?**

As mentioned before in this publication, **monthly breast self-exam** by women can pick up about 30% of breast cancers, both new ones and recurrences after breast conservation therapy. Others are too small to be felt, or palpated, but 85% of breast cancers can be detected with a mammogram.

The radiation dose from a modern mammogram is 0.2 centiGray, about the same as an ordinary chest X-ray. Worrisome findings on a mammogram include lots of little calcium deposits, called microcalcifications, especially in irregular or starburst patterns.

About 1/3 of these will represent cancer. Sometimes, a dominant mass may be felt in the breast, but the mammogram doesn't show anything. Any dominant mass must be biopsied (sampled) to rule out cancer! That's because 15% of even large cancers will remain invisible on a mammogram.

If a suspicious area is found, either on exam or mammogram, the National Cancer Institute recommends a 2 part approach. Firstly, a biopsy (sampling procedure) is done to confirm or deny cancer.

Then secondly, a surgery is performed to remove any cancer detected.

The quickest, easiest way to sample a suspicious area is called a fine needle aspiration in which a thin needle is placed into the tumor using radiographic guidance. Some cells are sucked up, or aspirated, and sent to a pathologist. This is a doctor who **specializes** in making diagnoses from tissue specimens.

This test is over 90% accurate at detecting cancer. If it is positive (that means cancer is found) then surgery is done. Either the entire breast is removed (called a **mastectomy**), or just the area of the tumor with a surrounding safety margin (called a **lumpectomy**).

The cancer removed is submitted for various tests, to classify it and see how likely it is to be aggressive.

These include the following Prognostic Factors:

**Grading the tumor:-** The pathologist looks at the cells in the tumor to see just how closely they resemble normal breast cells. He assigns a grade, called the Bloom-Richardson grade, from 1 to 3. A grade of 1 means that the tumor closely resembles normal breast, that is well-differentiated, and probably isn't very aggressive while a grade of 3 means the tumor looks very cancerous, that is poorly differentiated and is likely aggressive. A grade of 2 means moderately differentiated so is of intermediate behavior.

**Estrogen and Progesterone Receptor Studies** (**ER** and **PR** for short) look to see how likely the tumor is to respond to these female hormones. The chances of them being positive, **increases** with the age of the patient.

If both ER and PR are positive, the tumor is less aggressive and has an 80% chance of responding to anti-estrogen drugs like tamoxifen. If both are negative, there is only a 10% chance of response **Positive PR** with **Negative ER** is better than vice-versa.

**The DNA activity measurements of S-phase** (which tells how quickly the cells are dividing-- higher S-phase is more aggressive) and Ploidy which also tells how similar the cancer cells are genetically to normal breast cells. Diploid is normal and is better than aneuploid which is more cancerous. *Aneuploidy* is an abnormal number of chromosomes, and is a type of chromosome abnormality.

**Cathepsin D** -- is a cellular enzyme, a high level suggests positive lymph glands. It is an estrogen-induced lysosomal protease.

**Oncogenes** look genetically at the tumor, if the Breast Cancer (BCA-1) o a gene called HER-2/neu are increased, these tumors are **more aggressive.**

**The size of the tumor** - If it's less than 1 cm. across, 10 year survival is over 80% while if it's more than 7 cm. across, average 10 year survival is only 40%.

The larger the cancer grows locally (the higher the tumor burden), the more chance it has to spread to lymph nodes and to distant body areas. The pathologist also looks at the type of breast cells to classify the cancer as **ductal orlobular**, and to see if it invades through these ducts or lobules.

If the cancer invades (90% of them do) then it becomes necessary to do a second small operation, called an axillary lymph node sampling, which is not a therapeutic procedure, but merely diagnostic.

There procedure isn't done if the cancer isn't invasive (i.e. DCIS or LCIS).

If the axilla's lymph glands are negative (not involved) then 10 year survival is over 75%, while if more than 4 lymph nodes are positive (involved) 10 year average survival drops to only 25%.

The main point of checking the axilla is to see if chemotherapy will be necessary, if it is involved, this suggests that the cancer cells may have spread through the body, and chemotherapy will be necessary.

For any Locally Advanced or Inflammatory cancer, chemotherapy is essential.

**Other Standard Tests:** Include **bone-scan** where a small quantity of radioactive dye is injected into a vein and a special X-ray is then taken to see if the cancer has gone to bone.

**Breast cancer** has a **predilection to go to the bone**, where it may lie dormant for many years. A baseline scan is obtained for any invasive cancer, to make later scans easier to compare and interpret. If something is seen on a bone scan, it may or may not be cancer.

Old fractures, inflammation, or infections can make bone scans light up in those areas. The two ways of seeing if cancer is causing the increased uptake is to do a bone biopsy or another bone scan several months later to see if the area has progressed.

In practice, bone biopsy is difficult and may still miss an area of cancer spread, giving a false sense of security. Repeat scans, and the expertise of the radiologist in determining whether cancer is causing the abnormal bone scan are relied upon. Chest X-ray and Chest and Abdominal CT scans (Computerized Axial Tomography).

A contrast solution may be injected into an arm vein, which helps highlight blood vessels in a CT scan. **Insist upon having an _omnipaque_** brand or equivalent contrast used. According to GE, this contrast agent has been used in over 200 million patients worldwide.

Its indications include a broad range of intravascular diagnostic procedures such as coronary angiography, spinal cord imaging and body-cavity procedures.

It is more expensive, but also **more comfortable** and less likely to cause allergic reactions or kidney failure. These scans are obtained to help rule out spread, or metastasis of cancer to the lungs and liver.

CT scan of the Brain or Bone Marrow Biopsy are done only if there is suspicion that the cancer has spread to these organs, or if a bone-marrow transplant is considered. Routine blood tests of complete blood count (CBC) and chemistry panel (SMA) are obtained prior to any therapy.

**How is the Extensiveness of Breast Cancer Gauged?**
Like any cancer, the extensiveness of Breast Cancer is given by the **Stage**.

The American Joint Cancer Committee (AJCC) has stages given by Roman numerals:

**Stage 0** means the cancer does not invade, such as DCIS or LCIS
**Stage I** means the cancer is less than 1 inch across, and is invasive.
**Stage II** means the cancer is between 1 and 3 inches across, or the lymph glands in the axilla are involved (or both).
**Stage III** means that the cancer is greater than 3 inches across and the lymph glands in the axilla are involved and may even be hard and fixed.
**Stage IV** means that the cancer has spread to other organs, like bone or brain. This may be as little as a single lymph node involved above the collarbone (supraclavicular node) or as much as massive cancer spread (dissemination) throughout the body.

## What is the Survival of Breast Cancer?

This depends upon many factors, including the cancer type, grade and stage, the general condition of the patient, and the treatment(s) selected. The textbook figures are:

| Stage | 5-year Survival | 10-year Survival |
|-------|-----------------|------------------|
| 0     | 100%            | 98%              |
| I     | 90%             | 80%              |
| II    | 80%             | 70%              |
| III   | 50%             | 30%              |
| IV    | 20%             | 5%               |

It is crucial to note that many patients live many productive years with their cancer!

The figures given above include death from all causes, including heart attack, accidents, or a different cancer. Many patients with breast cancer are elderly and have other serious medical problems (comorbid conditions) leading to their demise.

**What are the types of Later Breast Cancer?**

There are **3 basic types**:

1) **Locally Advanced Breast Cancer** involves the local area of the breast and the axilla, and refers to a large but localized cancer.
2) **Metastatic Breast Cancer** means that the disease has spread to other body sites, such as the bone, liver, lung and brain.
3) **Inflammatory Breast Cancer** means that the drainage channels in the skin, called the dermal lymphatics, are obstructed by tumor-- this causes the breast to be hot, red and tender, and have a characteristic peau de orange (orange peel) texture.

**What is the Conventional Treatment for Later Breast Cancer?**

Treatment has historically consisted of surgery, radiation, chemotherapy, and hormones. The combination and sequence of these treatments has been refined over the past 2 decades.

Specifics of each of them, is now discussed with their historic results, followed by the **latest, effective** combination treatments and results.

Let us go back to the beginning now. **Surgery** was pioneered by Dr. Halstead in the 19th century-- At that time, before routine breast self-exam and mammograms, most cases were **later breast cancer** due to the time lapse before they came to medical attention.

Dr. Halstead felt that the more breast tissue and local muscle that could be removed, the better chance of curing the patient. He advocated radical mastectomy.

In this operation, the entire breast is removed, along with the underlying muscles of the chest wall (called the pectoralis muscles) and the lymph glands in the axilla.

Halstead believed that these lymph glands acted as trapping stations for the cancer, which would only spread through the body after the axilla was involved.

Thus it made sense to remove those lymph nodes before the cancer could spread from them. In the 1950's an even more radical operation, the extended radical mastectomy was done which was a **combination of a radical mastectomy** plus removing the lymph glands from under the breastbone (internal mammary nodes).

When the more drastic operations were not shown to increase cure, breast surgeons advocated modified radical mastectomy, where the major chest wall muscles were kept in place (which helps arm function) and the internal mammary lymph nodes were again not removed.

This remains the most common operation for breast removal today. Along with breast removal surgery, a new artificial breast may be constructed by sewing a back of gel material under the skin. Even a fake nipple can be formed.

**Side Effects of Surgery** include a standard operative death risk of 1-2%, infection risk of 10%, and possible arm weakness and swelling (called edema) with extensive surgery. The recovery period depends on the extent of surgery done. It is from weeks to months. Generally, tissues are 75% back to their normal strength 3 weeks after surgery.

The Results of surgery alone depended upon the **type** of Later Breast Cancer.

For **Locally Advanced** Breast Cancer, 5 year survival was about 40%.

For **Metastatic** Breast Cancer 5 year survival was 20%.

While for **Inflammatory** Breast Cancer, 5 year survival was a dismal 5%.

The reason for these poor survivals is that the cancer was already a systemic disease (cancer cells had spread through the body) before the surgery was performed, so the patients failed distantly after local surgical treatment.

We now move ahead to discuss what is being used in our generation. **Radiation Therapy** also called **Radiotherapy** in Great Britain, is currently almost always used for later cancer. It has been used alone for cancers that were too large to remove surgically, or for patients who couldn't tolerate surgery.

It used to be given by a radiologist who did X-rays, but is now prescribed by a specialized cancer doctor called a Radiation Oncologist.

Prior to starting treatment the patient is **Simulated**, which means they are placed on a fake treatment machine, the chest is exposed, and aligned with laser lights. Molds are made to be used during treatment. The patient receives small skin marks to guide the placement of treatment fields.

Which means that first the treatment area is marked out with pens and eventually with small permanent tattoos. A CT scan of the chest may be obtained, and the information from the simulation is put into a **treatment planning** computer.

**A plan** is generated, which tells how much radiation is going to the breast, axilla, and underlying normal tissue like lung. This plan is standardly publicationed by a Radiation Physicist (who has at least a Master's Degree and usually a Ph.D) to ensure its safety.

For locally advanced breast cancer it is common to use a three-field technique, that is the breast or chest wall is treated with 2 oblique radiation beams, while a third en-face field is aimed directly down to cover the area over the collarbone (clavicle) and axilla.

Special blocks are cut to protect sensitive normal tissues, such as the underlying lung, these are placed into the head of the treatment machine. The patient need only lie still on the hard table to receive their therapy due to the mold that was previously made of their torso.

Treatments are given Monday through Friday, taking only about 15 minutes per day for 6 - 7 weeks. The total dose of radiation is between 50 and 75 Gray (units of radiation) with the tumor area getting more dose than the regional lymphatics (the axilla and area above the collarbone).

X-ray verification films are taken each week or so, which tell only about the consistency of the patient's position; they do not tell anything about the cancer. Commonly, the last week of treatment is a boost to the actual tumor area, sparing the lesser involved areas.

The patient **does not get sick**, become radioactive or lose their hair. They can maintain a normal diet and most activities, like driving or taking occasional alcoholic beverages.

**Side effects** of local chest radiation are divided into acute and late effects. Acute effects occur during the treatment period, while late effects may occur months to years after treatment is complete.

Common acute effects include redness and tenderness in the treatment area, especially about the skin folds under the breast and in the armpit.

This starts occurring after about 2 weeks of treatments, and may progress to skin peeling, called desquamation.

Special salves, like **Acemannan** (a major carbohydrate fraction of **Aloe vera** gel, has been known to have antiviral and antitumoral activities), or **steroid creams** may reduce the irritation.

Patients are also usually mildly fatigued during the treatment period. Later effects of radiation include possible lung injury, called radiation pneumonitis, which is usually only detectable by chest X-ray and has no symptoms.

**Less than 10%** of these patients get symptoms of cough, shortness of breath, and fatigue-- which usually quickly respond to steroid medication. Skin reaction and heart or lung problems are greater if chemotherapy is also used.

**Very rarely** (<1%) patients may develop a severe syndrome of lung injury leading to death. Other later effects include arm swelling (especially if radiation is given after surgery) and very rarely second cancers developing in the swollen arm (lymphangiosarcoma) or in the irradiated lung (**especially in smokers**).

More commonly the radiation is well tolerated, the skin reaction subsides after finish of treatment, and the chest tissues become somewhat firmer and tougher (fibrotic). The skin may have small **bluish capillary markings**, and be lighter in color.

Ironically, some patients actually prefer the firmness of a breast which has been treated!

**Results of Radiation alone are similar to surgery, with 5 year average survival at 40% for locally advanced breast cancer, 20% for Metastatic breast cancer, and 5% for inflammatory breast cancer.

This again is because radiation, like surgery, only treats the local area of disease, while the cancer cells have already spread in the body.

**Chemotherapy** has **not been** conventionally used alone for treating breast cancer, but is extensively used in combination with other treatments as will be discussed.

Popular Chemotherapy drugs include Adriamycin (A), Cyclophosphamide (C), Methotrexate (M) and 5-Fluorouracil (5-FU or F). Taxol is a newer drug that will be discussed later. Combinations are frequently prescribed, such as CAF or CMF, usually given for six monthly cycles. A newer convenient regimen is AC times 4 -- that is just 2 drugs for 4 cycles.

The idea of Chemotherapy in Later Breast Cancer is two-fold-- to **shrink the tumor** and make it easier to remove or radiate, and to **kill** cancer cells which have escaped from the breast tumor, traveled through the bloodstream, and implanted elsewhere in the body.

These are called **micro-metastasis**, and although they cannot be detected with any current technology, since small numbers of cancer cells have spread from the **primary tumor** to other parts of the body and are too few to be picked up in a screening or diagnostic test. We know that they may be present and eventually grow into large tumors.

If they do, it is called **distant failure**, and this may be prevented with aggressive chemotherapy. Once the tumor burden of **metastatic cells is high** (i.e. they can be seen on scans) we cannot cure the patient (although they may live for many more productive years).

Chemotherapy **may** kill micro-metastasis and thus prevent the cancer from recurring, since it travels throughout the body (systemically). Chemotherapy is also useful for shrinking large local tumors and reducing the risk of local recurrence in the breast or chest after surgery. That is, it can help with local control.

Both effective local and distant control are mandatory if the patient is to be cured, utilizing multiple modalities (i.e. surgery, chemotherapy, radiation, hormones) for this purpose is called multi-modality therapy.

**Some Side Effects Of The Common Chemotherapeutic Agents Being Used In Therapy.**

1) **Adriamycin** can cause heart damage and the dose is limited to 500 mg/square meter of patient body surface area. It is common to get a heart scan called a MUGA test before giving Adriamycin.

It also causes greater skin redness and irritation (called a recall reaction) if radiation is given, even months later. It is a bright red liquid given only into the veins. Adriamycin chemotherapy is considered more radical than CMF, and is given when the tumor is aggressive.

2) **Cyclophosphamide** (also called Cytoxan) is derived from mustard gas and causes a lowering of blood counts. Drops in red-blood cell count cause anemia, with paleness and tiredness, drops in white-blood cell count lead to neutropenia which shows as infections and fevers, while a drop in platelet count leads to prolonged bleeding and easy bruising. Cyclophosphamide comes in a pill which is taken daily during each chemotherapy cycle.

2) **5-Fluorouracil (5-FU)** has its side effects on rapidly dividing cells in the body such as the lining of the intestines and also the bone

marrow. It can therefore lower blood counts, and cause mouth sores and diarrhea.

**Rarely**, 5-FU can cause skin peeling and nervous system symptoms. 5-FU is given into the veins either as individual injections on the first and eight day of each cycle (called bolus ) or as a constant drip of the drug during each cycle through a portable dose pack (called continuous infusion ).

**4) Methotrexate** has similar side effects to 5-FU, and can also cause a lowering of liver and kidney function. It comes as an intravenous injection, and can be given into the spinal fluid for the rare meningitis caused by spread of breast cancer to the central nervous system.

The Results of chemotherapy alone shows shrinkage in over 80% of tumors when it is given in combinations like CMF and CAF.

Practically speaking, however, it is difficult to completely obliterate breast cancer with chemotherapy alone, and the response may be short lived.

Cancer cells can develop resistance to chemotherapy. Therefore, it is **used in combination** with other treatments such as surgery and radiation, to increase its effectiveness.

Chemotherapy for breast cancer helps gain both local and distant control of disease-- and both are necessary for the patient to be cured.

**Hormonal Therapy** is extensively used in breast cancer, and is especially effective for **Estrogen Receptor Positive tumors, which** is the most frequent kind in women after their menopause.

It has been long noted that women who had their ovaries either removed surgically called oophorectomy or sterilized with radiation treatments often had a slowing of the progression of their breast cancer.

Instead of removing or radiating the ovaries, drugs have been developed which counteract the female hormones which can promote breast cancer growth. The **most common** anti-estrogen **drug** is **tamoxifen** (nolvadex) which is given as a 10 mg. tablet twice per day.

Since it also has some estrogen-like properties, it can cause an initial increase in bone pain, called a flare when it's first started. It commonly causes hot flashes and fatigue.

**Tamoxifen** also appears to **increase uterine cancer** in women who have kept their uterus. Breast cancer may respond to tamoxifen for many years, and then become resistant to it.

This usually shows up as progression on a bone scan indicating the cancer is growing again. Other hormonal drugs, called progestational agents such as medroxyprogesterone (megace) may then be effective.

It is given as a 40 mg. tab 4 times per day. The cancer cells may become resistant to progesterones also, after which male-sex hormones such as **Halotestin (Fluoxymesterone)** may be tried.

These **cause hair growth** and **increased muscle mass**, but may stymie the cancer for a while. There are many websites selling Halotestin for body builders. It is approximately 5 times as potent as **methyltestosterone**.

For later breast cancer, hormonal treatment is continued indefinitely, as long as it seems to hold the cancer at bay.

While **hormones don't cure** breast cancer, they can buy time; often patients with metastatic hormone responsive breast cancer live many years without evident progression.

### What is the Latest, Effective Therapy for Later Breast Cancer?

In general, the latest treatments use a combination of the above conventional treatments to reduce the chance that the cancer will come back. The specific treatment depends upon the type of later breast cancer.

### Locally Advanced Breast Cancer:

This is about 25% of new breast cancer cases. The newest treatments combines modified radical mastectomy, axillary lymph node dissection, **External Beam Radiation Treatment** to the chest wall to 60 Gray, and **chemotherapy** with either 6 cycles of CAF or 4 intense cycles of AC, follow by long-term **tamoxifen**.

Giving radiation had been controversial, but it is now definitely shown to lower local failure (which, when it occurs, is a painful, ugly process leading to a miserable death), and maybe up survival.

The survival benefit at 5-10 years combining all of the above treatments was shown in the Stockholm II trial and the Helsinki trial. Basically, both chest radiation and chemotherapy each benefit a given set of patients, and combining them, gives the additive advantages of both.

The Joint Center (at Harvard University) has shown that in patients with 4 or more positive lymph nodes in the axilla, radiation treatment reduces the risk of the breast cancer returning locally from 20% to 6%.

Let's cut to the chase, the **bottom line** of several studies is that patients with 4 or more involved lymph nodes and/or a breast tumor over 5 cm.

**should get Radiation Treatments** after their modified radical mastectomy, in addition to chemotherapy containing Adriamycin and long-term tamoxifen.

This regimen **increases** 10 year survival from just 30% to over 55% for locally advanced breast cancer. It is advisable to give the chemotherapy first since a decrease in tumor stage is seen in 30% of patients and at least some response is seen in 85%.

This helps tell how effective the chemotherapy is, and if it produces a complete response, the patient may then get radiation to the breast and local lymph node areas without a mastectomy!

This breast conservation for locally advanced breast cancer has been done by Dr. Hortobagyi at M.D. Anderson Cancer Center, with no compromise in survival.

**Bone Marrow Transplant:**

When patients have 10 or more positive lymph nodes in the axilla, autologous bone marrow transplant should be considered-- This means that the patient's own bone marrow is collected, and then very high doses of chemotherapy are used, to kill the cancer.

This dose of chemotherapy is so strong that it wipes out the remaining bone marrow, as well as the cancer cells (hopefully).

The patient would die of anemia and infection, except that the collected bone marrow can be re-injected into their veins (transplanted) where it finds its way back into the bones to grow into new blood-cell producing marrow.

For both **autologous transplants**, there are two basic ways that the blood-forming cells can be collected. The first and older technique is to harvest bone marrow from the iliac wing bones, located in the hip area.

The patient or matched donor is taken to the operating room and commonly put under general anesthesia.

About **50 punctures** are made with a special bone-boring needle into the bone above each buttock, and the marrow from this area sucked out (aspirated). There is no significant danger (besides anesthesia risk) to the patient, this marrow is expendable, but some scarring is common in the harvest area.

The **marrow** is stored in glass jars. Since breast cancer cells may have contaminated the bone marrow, it may be cleaned (purged) of breast cancer cells by using monoclonal antibodies (specially engineered immune proteins) against them. Research in this area is going on at the Dana Farber Cancer center. It is possible that directly injecting these monoclonal antibodies into the patient might help cure breast cancer.

New techniques have improved the success of purging, but it still remains a risk to give the patient back there their disease in the transplant.

The **second and newer** method is less invasive and does not take actual marrow, but instead stem cells circulating in the bloodstream. These **stem cells** can form new marrow, all of the crucial blood cells, and reconstitute the blood.

For stem-cell collection, the procedure is not called a Bone-Marrow transplant but instead a Peripheral Stem Cell Transplant. Since currently this procedure is used with the patient's own stem-cells, the full name is **Autologous Peripheral Stem Cell Transplant**.

For this, the patient comes in several times and has a needle (catheter) inserted into an arm vein. Blood is drawn out and processed through a special machine which collects stem cells, and then returns the residual blood back to the patient. The cells removed are centrifuged to remove the circulating stem cells, which are packaged and stored.

The next step for any Bone Marrow Transplant is for the patient's own marrow to be destroyed by chemotherapy (cytotoxic marrow ablation).

This is to annihilate the patient's breast cancer, and as a consequence destroys every other blood forming cell at the same time.

Sometimes, part of the preparative regimen for **Bone Marrow Transplant** is the addition of whole body radiation. For this, the patient is sent down to the Radiation Oncology Department for initial measurements of body thickness, and to make appropriate physics calculations.

During the **Marrow Ablation Phase** (and while receiving the chemotherapy) about 6 whole body radiation treatments are given over 3 days (so two treatments per day about 6 hours apart).

The patient, on a cart, is usually placed against a wall in the treatment room and the Linear Accelerator is turned on for about 10 minutes per treatment.

They are commonly treated from each side, with their arms at their sides to help lower the dose to the lungs.

A type of **plexiglass** scatter screen is placed between the patient and the machine, which helps **boost up** the dose to the skin. This is because leukemic cells can hide in the lower skin layers.

The actual radiation treatment is painless, and the patient is then returned to their room.

The side-effects of the preparative regimen for **Bone Marrow Transplant** are due to a killing of all the rapidly dividing cells in the body. The **side-effects** will depend on whether just chemotherapy is used, or whether whole-body radiation is added also.

The chemotherapy side-effects are the same as noted above for when these drugs are used a primary treatment, but for marrow ablation higher doses are given.

The dose is, in fact, **super-lethal**, since the patient will die if the bone marrow is not replaced. The first cells to disappear from the bloodstream are those with the shortest normal life-- white cells often only live 10 hours!

Next, the platelets, with an average life of 10 days, will disappear, and finally the red blood cells with an average life of 120 days.

If not replaced, we would expect to see in the following order. **Infection, Hemorrhage,** and thirdly, **Anemia** develop from the marrow ablative therapy.

In practice, the patient will not live long enough to develop anemia, first dying from infection and hemorrhage.

It takes a while for the re-infused bone marrow or stem cells to take, and start producing new blood cells.

This is a critical time for supportive transfusions and preventing infections. Epogen (erythropoetin) can help **boost the red blood cell**

**count** and Neupogen (GM-CSF) can boost the white cell count in this critical period.

**Results**: The initial complete response (CR) rate is as high as 65% (no detectable tumor remaining), and over 25% of patients may be cured of an otherwise fatal disease.

**Anti-rejection drugs** are not necessary since the patient's own bone marrow is being used, but there is still about a 10% chance of dying from complications of the procedure.

If you get a transplant, go to a hospital that does at least 50 per year. It unfortunately doesn't yet cure Metastatic breast cancer, although it may achieve prolonged remissions.

Locally Advanced is not a uniformly fatal disease-- aggressively treat it!

### Inflammatory Breast Cancer:

Used to have just 5% survival at 5 years-- The latest effective treatment is as given by Dr. Hortobagyi at M.D. Anderson Cancer Center and Dr. Fowble at the University of Pennsylvania.

It is induction chemotherapy with CAF and BCG (an immune stimulant).

Patients who have a complete response (no evidence of tumor) get Radiation Therapy to the breast and local lymph nodes to 50 Gray, plus a boost to the actual tumor site (so the total radiation dose to the tumor is about 70 Gray).

If there is a partial or no response to chemotherapy, a modified radical mastectomy is done with radiation therapy to 50 Gray given to the chest wall and local lymph nodes.

**\*\*Results improve** to 65% survival at 5 years with no sign of disease! Furthermore, up to 30% of women (those completely responding to chamois.) **keep their breast**!

**Metastatic Breast Cancer:**

Still remains one of the most difficult cancers to treat. Unfortunately, no current therapy definitely cures breast cancer which has obviously spread to the bone and other organs.

Naturally, is it important to be sure that the cancer actually has spread, and that the abnormal uptake seen on a bone scan is really cancer.

This is accomplished with serial bone scans every several months to see how the area is changing.

We cannot definitely say that no one has ever been cured with metastatic breast cancer, since patients may have had unrecognized metastasis at diagnosis, gotten intensive chemotherapy or even bone marrow transplant, and been cured.

The rate of total remission (no evident cancer remaining) in bone marrow transplant patients with metastatic breast cancer is as high as 50%, but many of these patients had not had prior therapy. Mostly, chemotherapy has been started only to treat specific symptoms.

The **most effective** chemotherapy contains **Adriamycin** (Doxorubicin), it is about 18% **more effective** than chemotherapy without it.

In fact, Adriamycin alone is as effective as other combination regimens of multiple drugs. Often Adriamycin is reserved until other agents fail, since there is no good third line chemotherapy for metastatic breast cancer.

Patients with metastasis to the soft tissue (e.g. muscle or fat) are most likely to respond to chemotherapy, patients with metastasis to lung or liver least likely, and patients with bone metastasis in the middle.

Giving **salvage chemotherapy** for patients with isolated bone metastasis has produced occasional complete remissions lasting 5 years or more.

The addition of the **biochemical modifier leucovorin** along with 5-FU has shown promising results as second line therapy in breast cancer, as it has in primary colon cancer.

If a patient responds to chemotherapy, the bone metastasis will slowly disappear (recalcification will occur) and the average response lasts 18 months.

The main problem with chemotherapy in metastatic breast cancer is that many patients have previously been treated, and so developed resistance to the drugs.

One advantage of having a bone metastasis is having something to follow. If no response occurs after 3 cycles of chemotherapy, other non-cross resistant agents should be tried.

The duration of remission is increased if effective chemotherapy is given continuously, as opposed to the usual 6 cycles.

However, it has not been proven that this continued maintenance chemotherapy improves survival; and the patient must tolerate the side effects of hair loss, nausea and decreased blood counts.

**Taxol** has about a 30% response rate in breast cancer which has failed other therapies, but causes nausea, flu-like symptoms, and lowered blood counts. It is our most effective third line agent available for breast or ovarian cancer.

In **hormone-responsive patients**, the chemotherapy can be combined with hormones. Metastatic breast cancer is thought to contain different subgroups or clones of cells; some will be responsive to chemotherapy but not hormones, and vice-versa.

Thus the chance of a long term remission **is greater** if chemotherapy is **added** to **hormonal therapy**, in **both premenstrual** and **postmenopausal** patients with hormone receptors.

**Hormone Treatment** alone is aimed at slowing the cancer and improving quality of life. It is not considered curative, but some patients have had sustained complete remissions lasting many years with hormones alone.

Firstly, hormones work primarily in patients with hormone responsive (ER/PR positive) tumors. If both of these receptors are absent, the chance of hormones working is only 10%. However, if both ER and PR are present, the chance increases to around 70%.

The average duration of response with a hormone is 18 months, after which the cancer progresses. Then a second line hormone is used, and then a third line one.

The chance for response will decrease with each successive hormone tried. Thus many doctors don't try fourth line hormones.

However, if hormone receptors are present but one agent doesn't work, the chance of responding to a different one is still excellent in the hormone responsive patient.

The first hormonal manipulation encouraged for hormone responsive patients with breast cancer metastasis is having their ovaries removed (oophorectomy) or **radiated to destroy** them.

This alone has held the cancer at bay for many years in occasional patients. Giving hormones (first tamoxifen, then megace, or goseralin acetate, then halotestin) can often slow the progress of the cancer significantly.

Hormones can be taken as pills, or often as deep muscle depot injections each month. Patients may live for many years with Metastatic breast cancer, and symptoms are treated as they arise. It may be a very indolent disease.

However, symptoms should be treated aggressively, and some are even medical emergencies. When breast cancer is the most advanced type with distant disease spread through the body, the objective is no longer cure but palliation (meaning relief of pain and other symptoms).

The patient would be made as comfortable as possible, and narcotic medicines like **morphine** should **never be withheld** for fear of causing addiction.

Using **Fentanyl Patches** applied to the skin **helps** give a continuous amount of narcotic, eliminating the problems of forgotten doses, loss of narcotics, and smoothing out the dosing for less disturbing highs and lows.

**Radiation Treatment** can help relief local symptoms (such as skin involvement), bleeding, and bone pain in over 80% of patients.

It is helpful if bones have become weakened from cancer invasion, and have fractured (pathological fracture) or are in danger of doing so.

Radiation Therapy centers with hyperthermia can use this newer technology to heat an area of skin metastasis, and then give the radiation treatment.

This is very effective for reducing unsightly skin spread more quickly and effectively than standard radiation treatment.

**Hyperthermia** is now approved in the U.S. for treatment of Breast cancer recurrence, and it is covered by insurance. This is how heat therapy works: Heat results when atoms and molecules vibrate and move around at a higher rate or frequency.

The body uses its own internally generated heat to protect itself from viruses, bacteria, and other harmful substances. A fever is the body's highly evolved attempt to destroy invading organisms and to sweat impurities out through the skin.

**Fever** is an **effective natural process** of curing disease and restoring health; heat therapy, or hyperthermia, represents a way to create fever to call out this natural healing process.

Cancer cells are more heat sensitive than normal tissues and are more easily killed by heating. Localizing the heat is important, since one cannot raise the whole-body temperature to 42' C or 43' C without lethal consequences.

Another strategy is to raise the whole-body temperature in a more moderate way, from 37' C to 40' C (98.6' F to 104' F). This may be performed by using whole-body wet wraps, saunas, and hot baths.

When used in combination with taking ginseng or other substances that increase the effect of heat, it can be of value in cancer treatment.

**Hyperthermia** is also useful for decreasing the dose needed to control massive local disease invading the chest wall, with its attendant problems of pain, oozing fluid and infection. You'll find a **list of Doctors** who give this therapy at the **end of this publication**.

**Radiation** is utilized for reducing the symptoms, and even extending survival, in patients with spread to the brain.

Sometimes radiation therapy is used as an emergency measure when the cancer spreads to the spinal column and threatens to cause paralysis by pressing upon the spinal cord.

**Any patient with breast cancer** who experiences new weakness of the extremities, **numbness**, or **loss** of **bowel** or **bladder function** must be brought into the <u>**Emergency Room immediately**</u> to see whether the tumor is compressing the spinal cord causing these symptoms.

Up to 60% of new back pain in a cancer patient is caused by spread of cancer there. The patient is given a painless Magnetic Resonance Imaging (MRI) scan to check for epidural spinal cord compression.

If this is caught early, and treatment is given, permanent paralysis may be prevented. It is unfortunately uncommon to reverse symptoms of paralysis once they have set it.

However, so quick recognition is essential. As mentioned, radiation treatment can be very helpful for metastatic breast cancer. A relatively **new method** of radiation for spread to the brain (one of the most common areas of spread) is **Stereotactic Radiosurgery.**

Where multiple beams of convergent radiation are aimed onto the area(s) of spread in brain, or in a single painless session in one afternoon. This is usually followed by conventional **External Beam Radiation.**

The **advantage** of **Stereotactic Radiosurgery** is that it can give a **very high dose** of radiation to areas of brain metastasis, and possibly enhance survival for these patients, without the risk of an open brain surgery from a neurosurgeon.

We have available on our web site www.cancergroup.com a full publications written on **In-Depth Radiation Therapy** and an In-Depth publication on **Symptom Relief.**

Other options for patients in severe pain for multiple areas of spread to bone include hemi-body radiation, and strontium-89. Hemi-Body radiation uses a low dose (6 to 8 Gray) in a single treatment to the upper or lower body to treat multiple areas of bony involvement; some anti-nauseants are usually necessary and it lowers blood counts.

It is over **90% effective for pain relief** lasting an average of 6 months. Strontium-89 is an injected radioisotope that goes through the bloodstream to all bony areas, and is especially attracted to cancerous areas. It also lowers blood counts but is very effective at palliating pain.

It can only be done once. If no relief is gotten from medications or radiation, neurosurgical techniques to cut sensory nerves can usually afford relief, to this small population of patients.

The **most common cause of death in breast cancer** spread to bone is increased blood calcium, which manifests as **hypercalcemia**, an elevated calcium level in the blood.

Studies have found that injectable **Gallium Nitrate** is the **most effective** drug for combating this even better than **Etidronate** and it may prolong the patient's life.

**What Can I Do If My Cancer Comes Back?**

If the cancer recurs in the breast after breast conservation therapy (about a 10% chance) then Mastectomy is advocated, and has a 5 year survival of up to 85%.

Dr. Kurtz in St. Louis and others will now do another local excision surgery (lumpectomy) if the new tumor is small, located within the breast, and occurs at least 5 years after the first treatment was given.

If the cancer comes back before 5 years, there is a decreased survival rate, but if it comes back after 5 years, survival doesn't appear to be any worse!

Obviously, it makes a difference whether the failure is local or distant - but even those found to have distant metastasis to bone (the most common site) often live many years with appropriate therapy.

For local failure only, the latest studies show the breast may still be saved, after a small recurrence.

No further chemotherapy is given for small, non-invasive recurrent breast cancer, and no further radiation is given either - just surgery alone is enough.

Careful monitoring with breast exam and yearly mammograms is crucial in the patient who had had breast cancer, of either both breasts (if breast conservation therapy was performed) or the remaining breast if a mastectomy was done.

**In Conclusion:**

The patient with newly diagnosed breast cancer should not rely upon any single therapy, such as a pill or ray, but instead should use a **combination** approach to maximize the chance for success.

Specifically, besides the conventional medical therapies mentioned above, consider the use of a non-toxic, not over-expensive alternative therapy you can believe in.

We have available on our web site a publication for Alternative Therapies on Breast Cancer. Also, a program of spiritual renewal, mind over cancer, nutritional therapy and exercise is appropriate.

Keep the most **positive attitude** possible. Research has shown this to be an important factor in cancer survival.

Using a true **multi-modality** approach will give the confidence that you have done everything possible for a happy outcome, and will anyway improve quality of life, If the patient is willing to subject themselves to medical research. Advances in the past two decades make it more likely for the patient with later breast cancer to live longer and more comfortable lives than in the past, and have new cause to hope for tomorrow.

## LATEST CLINICAL TRIALS

Clinical Trials often have specific enrollment criteria, however, one cannot select which treatment (which arm of the study) they wish participate in.

Thus, one loses control of their treatment when entering a Clinical Trial. NSABP trials are well designed and will not shirk a patient from basic established therapy; they are now to fine-tune the treatments.

**Impact of 18F-FDG PET-CT Versus Conventional Staging in the Management of Patients Presenting With Clinical Stage III Breast Cancer (PET ABC).**

Sponsor: Ontario Clinical Oncology Group (OCOG)

Condition Intervention:- Stage III Breast Cancer (T0N2, T1N2, T2N2, T3N1, 2 or T4) - Stage IIb Breast Cancer (T3N0)

**Primary Outcome Measures:-** Proportion of patients upstaged to Stage IV disease [Time Frame: Within 30 days from date of randomization] Proportion of patients upstaged to Stage IV disease as a result of the imaging study, between the groups

**Secondary Outcome Measures:-** Proportion of patients who receive multimodal therapy of curative intent [Time Frame: Within 12 months from date of randomization].

Number of additional tests, such as imaging and biopsy, resulting from findings of study imaging [Time Frame: Within 12 months from date of randomization].

Prognostic ability of PET SUV of the primary lesion on the pathological response rate to neo-adjuvant chemotherapy [Time Frame: Within 12 months from date of randomization].

Disease Free Survival [Time Frame: From date of randomization to date of event, assessed up to 5 years].

Objectively defined local or distance recurrence or death.

Overall Survival [Time Frame: From date of randomization to date of event, assessed up to 5 years] Defined by all-cause mortality.

Incremental economic analysis comparing the costs and outcomes of the treatment arms [Time Frame: Within 5 years from date of randomization].

Utility values will be collected using the EQ-5D Health Utility Questionnaire and converted to quality adjusted life years (QALYs) by considering Overall Survival. Direct medical resources (i.e. tests, complications, hospitalizations, clinic visits, emergency dept., etc.) will be obtained. Costs ($CAN2016) for each resource identified and utilized will be determined. Finally, an incremental cost-utility analysis will be calculated comparing the 2 randomized arms to generate an incremental cost per QALY outcome.

Estimated Enrollment: 370
Study Start Date: December 2016
Estimated Study Completion Date: December 2023
Estimated Primary Completion Date: December 2019 (Final data collection date for primary outcome measure)

## Eligibility

Ages Eligible for Study: 18 Years and older (Adult, Senior)
Sexes Eligible for Study: All
Accepts Healthy Volunteers: No
Criteria

## Inclusion Criteria:

Women (or men) with histological evidence of breast cancer for whom potentially curative treatment is planned.

Based on clinical information (physical exam, imaging):
Stage III breast cancer (T0N2, T1N2, T2N2, T3N1, 2 or T4), or

Stage IIb breast cancer (T3N0), Note: T2N1 is not eligible

Considered for combined modality therapy (surgical resection, chemotherapy, radiotherapy) of curative intent.

## Exclusion Criteria:

Age < 18 years,
ECOG performance status > and = 3,
Prior systemic therapy (e.g. neo-adjuvant chemotherapy or hormonal therapy) for current breast cancer,
Previous staging investigations for current breast cancer,
Breast cancer with primary histological subtypes other than ductal or lobular (Note: Patients with mixed disease will be eligible for randomization),
Clinical suspicion of metastatic disease,
Relative contraindications to PET (e.g. uncontrolled diabetes (i.e. inability to decrease serum glucose below 10.2 mmol/L), claustrophobia, inability to be still for 30 minutes),
Inability to lie supine for imaging with PET-CT,
Inability to undergo CT because of known allergy to contrast,
History of another invasive malignancy within the previous two years (exception of non-melanoma skin cancer) or a synchronous primary cancer, including a synchronous contralateral breast cancer (Note: Patients found to have a contralateral breast cancer on study imaging following randomization will remain in the study),
Known pregnancy or lactating female,
Inability to complete the study or required follow-up.

## Contacts and Locations:-

Juravinski Cancer Centre        Recruiting

Hamilton, Ontario, Canada, L8V 5C2

Contact: Helen Shing, RN   905-387-9711   shing@hhsc.ca
Principal Investigator: Bindi Dhesy, MD

Thunder Bay Regional Health Sciences Centre
Thunder Bay, Ontario, Canada, P7B 6V4
Contact: Lori Moon, RN   807-684-7226   moonl@tbh.net
Principal Investigator: Adrien Chan, MD

---

**Trial to Compare the Efficacy and Safety of Pegfilgrastim Biosimilar in Subjects With High Risk Stage Breast Cancer Receiving Chemotherapy.**

**Purpose:-** This is a Phase III, randomised, assessor-blind, parallel group, multicentre trial. At least 180 adult subjects with high-risk Stage II or Stage III / IV breast cancer will be randomised (1:1) to receive either Eurofarma's pegfilgrastim (n = 90) or Neulastim (n = 90) in 8 to 10 sites in Brazil. Subjects will undergo a maximum of 4 cycles of myelosuppressive chemotherapy (21 days per cycle).

Estimated Enrollment:                 180
Study Start Date:                     April 2017
Estimated Study Completion Date:      October 2019
Estimated Primary Completion Date:    October 2019 (Final data collection date for primary outcome measure).

**Eligibility:-**

Ages Eligible for Study:     18 Years and older   (Adult, Senior)
Sexes Eligible for Study:    All

**Inclusion Criteria:**

Signed written informed consent.
Males or females ≥ 18 years of age (at the time of signing consent).

Breast cancer high-risk Stage II, or Stage III, or Stage IV (classification according to American Joint Committee on Cancer).
Eligible to receive 4 cycles of docetaxel and doxorubicin combination CTX for the treatment of high-risk stage II, III, or IV breast cancer.
CTX-naïve.
ECOG performance status ≤ 2.

**Adequate bone marrow function:**
Leucocyte count < 50 x 109/L.
ANC ≥ 1.5 x 109/L.
Platelet count ≥ 100 x 109/L.
Haemoglobin ≥ 10 x g/dL.
Left Ventricular Ejection Fraction (LVEF) ≥ 50% by echocardiography or equivalent method (e.g. Multi Gated Acquisition scan) within 4 weeks prior to administration of the first dose of trial medication.

Alanine aminotransferase and aspartate aminotransferase < 2.5 x upper limit of normal (ULN), alkaline phosphatase < 5 x ULN.
Total bilirubin ≤ ULN.
Creatinine ≤ 1.5 x ULN.

Female subjects of childbearing potential must have a negative serum pregnancy test within 14 days of first dose of trial treatment and agree to use highly effective contraception (e.g. hormonal contraception or intra-uterine device [which should be established prior to the start of the trial], plus usage by at least 1 of the partners of an additional spermicide-containing barrier method of contraception) from 2 weeks prior to administration of the first dose of trial medication until trial completion, and for 30 days after the last dose of trial drug.

Female subjects of non-childbearing potential must have a documented tubal ligation or hysterectomy; or postmenopausal defined as 12 months of spontaneous amenorrhea. A male subject with a female partner of childbearing potential must have either had a prior vasectomy or agree to use effective contraception from 2 weeks prior to administration of the first dose of trial medication until trial completion, and for 30 days after the last dose of trial drug.

## Exclusion Criteria:

Severe chronic neutropenia.
History of chronic myeloid leukemia or myelodysplastic syndrome.
History of sickle cell disease.
Previous or concurrent malignancy except non-invasive non-melanomatous skin cancer, in situ carcinoma of the cervix, or other solid Tumor treated curatively, and without evidence of recurrence for at least 10 years prior to trial entry.

Active uncontrolled infection.
Known human immunodeficiency virus seropositivity; active hepatitis B or hepatitis C at the Screening Visit.
Clinically significant impairment of LVEF.
Severe valvular heart disease, myocardial infarction, heart failure, unstable angina pectoris, uncontrolled hypertension, or uncontrolled arrhythmias within 6 months of the Screening.

## Visit
Significant neurologic or psychiatric disorders including psychotic disorders, dementia, or seizures that would prohibit the understanding and giving of informed consent.

Concurrent or prior radiotherapy within 4 weeks of the Screening Visit. Tumor surgery within 4 weeks prior to administration of the first dose of trial medication.

Concurrent or prior anti-cancer treatment for breast cancer such as endocrine therapy, immunotherapy, monoclonal antibodies, and/or biological therapy.

Concurrent prophylactic antibiotics or antibiotic treatment within 72 hours before CTX.

Prior bone marrow or stem cell transplant.

Previous therapy with any recombinant human granulocyte colony stimulating factor (G CSF) product.

Known hypersensitivity to docetaxel, doxorubicin, pegfilgrastim, filgrastim, Escherichia coli proteins, or any of the excipients used in the trial medication.

Treatment with lithium at randomization.
Known **controlled drug addiction**, including alcoholism.

Participation in a clinical trial within 30 days prior to the Screening Visit.

Pregnant or nursing women, women planning to become pregnant, or women of childbearing potential who do not agree to use highly effective contraception (e.g. hormonal contraception or intra-uterine device [which should be established prior to the start of the trial], plus usage by at least 1 of the partners of an additional spermicide-containing barrier method of contraception) from 2 weeks prior to administration of the first dose of trial medication until trial completion and for 30 days after the last dose of trial drug.

Male subjects with a female partner of childbearing potential who have not had a prior vasectomy and do not agree to use highly effective contraception from 2 weeks prior to administration of the first dose of trial medication until trial completion and for 30 days after the last dose of trial drug.

Any severe concurrent disease or condition, which in the judgment of the Investigator would make the subject inappropriate for trial participation. Peripheral neuropathy (sensory/motor) Grade 2 or higher (CTCAE, Version 4.03).

Chronic use of corticosteroids.

**Contacts and Locations:-**

Contact: Suely K Inoue, Pharm D +551150908410
        suely.inoue@eurofarma.com.br
Contact: Cassiano O Berto, Pharm D +551150908412
        cassiano.berto@eurofarma.com.br

---

## A Trail of Neoadjuvant Endostar in Combination With Chemotherapy in Breast Cancer (TENDENCY).

**Purpose:-**

This trial is designed to study the efficacy and safety of neoadjuvant docetaxel, epirubicin in combination with cyclophosphamide(DEC) plus human recombinant endostatin (endostar) for breast cancer patients. The hypothesis of this protocol is that the combined an active angiogenesis agent to chemotherapy could enhance the pathological response rate and further benefit breast cancer patients.

Estimated Enrollment:             300
Study Start Date:                 August 2018
Estimated Study Completion Date:  December 2021
Estimated Primary Completion Date: August 2020 (Final data collection date for primary outcome measure).

**Eligibility:-**

Ages Eligible for Study:    18 Years to 70 Years  (Adult, Senior)
Sexes Eligible for Study:   Female

## Inclusion Criteria:

Histologically confirmed invasive breast cancer (core needle biopsy for breast cancer diagnosis and fine needle aspiration for lymph node metastasis diagnosis).

Age 18-70
No evidence of distant metastasis
No previous therapy
Normal hematologic function
No abnormality of renal or liver function
Written informed consent

## Exclusion Criteria:

With allergic constitution or possible allergic reflection to drugs to be used in this study.

Any concurrent uncontrolled medical or psychiatric disorder.
History of severe heart diseases, including congestive heart failure, unstable angina, uncontrolled arrhythmia, myocardial infarction, uncontrolled high blood pressure, or heart valve disease.
Being pregnant or nursing.

**For More Information:-** Yunjiang Liu, M.D, Chief Physician of Breast Cancer Dept, Vice-President of Hebei Medical University Fourth Hospital, Hebei Medical University Fourth Hospital.

## Vaccine Therapy in Treating Patients With HER2-Negative Stage III-IV Breast Cancer.

**Purpose:-** This phase I trial studies the side effects and best dose of multiantigen deoxyribonucleic acid (DNA) plasmid-based vaccine in treating patients with human epidermal growth factor receptor 2 (HER2)-negative stage III-IV breast cancer. Multiantigen DNA plasmid-based vaccine may target immunogenic proteins expressed in breast cancer stem cells which are the component of breast cancer that is resistant to chemotherapy and has the ability to spread. Vaccines made from DNA may help the body build an effective immune response to kill tumor cells.

**Condition:-**
HER2/Neu Negative
Recurrent Breast Carcinoma
Stage IIIA Breast Cancer
Stage IIIB Breast Cancer
Stage IIIC Breast Cancer
Stage IV Breast Cancer
Stage III Breast Cancer

**Primary Outcome Measures:**

Immunologic efficacy defined as achievement of a statistically significant increase in Th1 cell immunity for at least 50% of the immunizing antigens as compared to baseline [Time Frame: Up to 5 years]
Incidence of toxicity per Cancer Therapy Evaluation Program Common Terminology Criteria for Adverse Events version 4.0 [Time Frame: Up to 1 month after last vaccine]

Ages Eligible for Study:        18 Years and older   (Adult, Senior).

**Inclusion Criteria:**

Patients with stage III-IV HER2 negative breast cancer treated with primary or salvage therapy and now have:
No evidence of disease (NED), or Stable bone only disease.
Patients who have completed standard of care and recovered with mild to no residual toxicity from recent therapy.

Patients must be at least 28 days post cytotoxic chemotherapy, and/or monoclonal antibody therapy (excluding bone-directed therapy), prior to enrollment.

Patients must be at least 28 days post systemic steroids prior to enrollment.

Patients on bisphosphonates, denosumab, and/or endocrine therapy are eligible.

Patients must have Eastern Cooperative Oncology Group (ECOG) performance status score of =< 1.

Patients must have recovered from major infections and/or surgical procedures, and in the opinion of the investigator, not have any significant active concurrent medical illnesses precluding protocol treatment.

Estimated life expectancy of more than >6 months.
White blood cells (WBC) >= 3000/mm^3.
Lymphocyte count >= 800/mm^3.
Platelet count >= 75000/mm^3.
Hemoglobin (Hgb) >= 10 g/dl.
Serum creatinine =< 1.2 mg/dl when adjusted for body surface area (BSA) or creatinine clearance > 60 ml/min.
Total bilirubin =< 1.5 mg/dl.
Aspartate aminotransferase (AST)/serum glutamic oxaloacetic transaminase (SGOT) =< 2 times upper limit of normal (ULN).
Blood glucose < 1.5 ULN.
All patients who are having sex that can lead to pregnancy must agree to contraception for the duration of study.

**Exclusion Criteria:**

Patients with any of the following cardiac conditions:
Symptomatic restrictive cardiomyopathy.
Unstable angina within 4 months prior to enrollment.
New York Heart Association functional class III-IV heart failure on active treatment.

Symptomatic pericardial effusion.
Patients at risk for gastrointestinal bleeding (example: peptic ulcer disease, prolonged daily non-steroidal anti-inflammatory use).
Patients with any seizure disorder.

Patients with any contraindication to receiving rhuGM-CSF based products.

Patients with any clinically significant autoimmune disease uncontrolled with treatment.

Patients who are simultaneously enrolled in any other treatment study.
Patients who are pregnant or breastfeeding.

**Recruiting:-** Fred Hutch/University of Washington Cancer Consortium.

Seattle, Washington, United States, 98109.
Contact: Mary L. Disis   206-616-1823   ndisis@u.washington.edu -
Principal Investigator: Mary L. Disis.

**A Multicenter Study of Clinical Epidemiology of Breast Cancer in Shaanxi Province of China.**

The purpose of the study is to study the epidemic features and diagnosis of female breast cancer, especially the diagnosis and treatment of breast cancer. The disease-free survival (DFS) and the total survival time(OS) of the breast cancer patients will also be studied.

## Detailed Description:

The study is a multicentric, retrospective clinical study based on the hospital. The target number of cases are X patients who are eligible for breast cancer after radical mastectomy. To collect the clinicopathological data and treatment data of the breast cancer patients and do the follow-up visit of all the patients who are included in the study.

## Eligibility:-

| | |
|---|---|
| Ages Eligible for Study: | Child, Adult, Senior |
| Sexes Eligible for Study: | Female |
| Accepts Healthy Volunteers: | No |
| Sampling Method: | Non-Probability Sample |

**Contact:** Yu Ren, MD,PhD    13700222161    renyyyyy@126.com

## Genomic Testing for Primary Breast Cancer.

## Purpose:-

The goal of this research study is find out if researchers can use genetic testing on tumor samples to predict if tumors will respond to breast cancer treatments. The tumor sample will be tested to learn if certain genes are activated (turned on) in the tumor. Researchers hope that the activation of these genes may predict if the tumor will be sensitive or resistant to routine breast cancer treatments, such as chemotherapy or hormonal therapy.

**Eligibility:-**

| | |
|---|---|
| Ages Eligible for Study: | 18 Years and older   (Adult, Senior) |
| Sexes Eligible for Study: | Female |
| Accepts Healthy Volunteers: | No |
| Sampling Method: | Probability Sample |
| Study Population | |

Breast cancer patients from UT MD Anderson Cancer Center in Houston, **Texas**

## Inclusion Criteria:

1. The patient can undergo biopsy or surgery of a primary tumor site for suspected or proven invasive breast cancer of clinical Stage I to III; stage IV patients will be allowed and included in the feasibility assessment, but will not be included in outcomes analysis for secondary objectives 1.2.4, 1.2.5 and 1.2.6.
2. The clinical or radiologic primary tumor size is at least 1 cm diameter.

**Locations:-** University of Texas MD Anderson Cancer Center.
**Recruiting:-** Houston, Texas, United States, 77030.
**Principal Investigator:-** Stacy Moulder, MD.
**Phone:-** 713-792-2817 or Fax: 713-794-4385
**Email:-** smoulder@mdanderson.org

---

## A Study to Evaluate the Accuracy of a Breast Cancer Locator (BCL) in Patients With Palpable Cancers.

**Purpose:-** In this study, the investigators will enroll women with palpable cancers to assess the accuracy of the Breast Cancer Locator (BCL) and concomitant procedure as a vehicle to optimize and validate the approach in surgical cases where the new device will not substantially alter or modify the standard-of-care procedure before initiating an evaluative trial of the BCL in non-palpable breast cancer cases.

**Detailed Description:** The investigators propose to test whether the Breast Cancer Locator (BCL) accurately defines the edges of the cancer. Twenty patients with palpable invasive breast cancer will undergo preoperative supine MRI, creation of a BCL, and breast conserving surgery using the BCL as an adjunct to palpation-guided tumor resection. Participants will also have the tumor position on their skin localized with the supine MR/optical scan/tracker method. The primary objective is to measure the distance from the center of the spots made by the BCL to the cancer edges.

**Locations:-** United States, New Hampshire
Dartmouth Hitchcock Medical Center   Recruiting
Lebanon, New Hampshire, United States, 03756
**Contact:-** Richard J Barth, MD   800-639-6918
Richard.J.Barth@hitchcock.org
**Contact:-** Research Nurse   800-639-6918
cancer.research.nurse@dartmouth.edu

---

**Vaccination With Autologous Breast Cancer Cells Engineered to Secrete Granulocyte-Macrophage Colony-Stimulating Factor (GM-CSF) in Metastatic Breast Cancer Patients.**

**Purpose:-** The purpose of this trial is to test the safety of a vaccine made from a patient's own breast cancer cells, and determine if this vaccine will delay or stop the growth of the cancer. The vaccine is made by genetically modifying a patient's own tumor cells to secrete granulocyte-macrophage colony-stimulating factor (GM-CSF) to activate the immune response.

**Primary Outcome Measures:-** To determine the doses of lethally irradiated, autologous breast cancer cells engineered by adenoviral

mediated gene transfer to secrete GM-CSF that can be manufactured in patients with metastatic breast cancer [Time Frame: 3 years].
To determine the safety and biologic activity of this vaccination in metastatic breast cancer patients [Time Frame: 3 years].
**Principal Investigator:** Beth Overmoyer, MD.
**Dana-Farber Cancer Institute**
**Office phone:** 617-632-3800
**Appointment phone:** 617-632-2175

---

**Autologous Vaccination With Lethally Irradiated, Autologous Breast Cancer Cells Engineered to Secrete GM-CSF in Women With Operable Breast Cancer.**

**Detailed Description:-** After the patient has given their consent to participate in the trial, a series of tests will be performed to determine if the patient is eligible. These tests may take place up to 21 days before the surgery to remove a tumor sample or cancer-containing fluid, which will be used to create the vaccines.

The tumor cells or fluid is then brought to a special, certified laboratory where the vaccine is made. Specially trained laboratory technicians then use a method known as adenoviral mediated gene transfer, which adds a new gene to the cancer cells. This gene causes the cells to make GM-CSF, a powerful hormone that stimulates the immune system. The cells are then given radiation so that they will not grow.

Participants will start receiving vaccine on day 1, 8, 15, 29, and then every two weeks until the supply of vaccine has run out. The amount of the vaccine depends upon the total amount of cells that are obtained from the breast cancer tumor or fluid. Each time the patient is vaccinated, they will be given injections that will be placed underneath the skin. A different place will be used for each injection. If there are enough cells from the patient's tumor sample, the patient will be given an injection of non-transduced irradiated cells (the gene was not added).

These cells will help to measure how the patient's immune system is reacting to the tumor cells. This is called Delayed-Type Hypersensitivity (DTH).

With vaccine #1 and #5, the patient will also receive a DTH injection. Two to three days after the vaccine and DTH injection, skin biopsies will be taken of both sites. At week 10 in the study treatment, or earlier if necessary, the patient will have a chest, abdomen, and pelvic CT scan to determine if the vaccine therapy has had an effect on their disease. A brain MRI will be performed if there were any abnormalities on the first brain MRI or if new symptoms have developed.

Patients may participate in this study until one of the following happens: All vaccine created from the tumor has been given to the patient; the patient's disease worsens; the patient experiences an unacceptable and/or harmful side effect; the patient is unable to follow the study plan; or the patient's doctor feels it is no longer in the best interest of the patient to continue.

**Locations:-** United States, Massachusetts.
**Brigham and Women's Hospital** - Boston, Massachusetts, United States, 02115.
**Phone:-** 617-732-5500.

**Dana-Farber Cancer Institute** - Boston, Massachusetts, United States, 02115.
Phone:- 877-442-3324.
Main number:- 617-632-3000
Toll-free:- 866-408-DFCI (3324).
**Principal Investigator:** Beth Overmoyer, MD.

**Dana-Farber Cancer Institute**
**Office phone:** 617-632-3800
**Appointment phone:** 617-632-2175.

**Study on SBRT for Inoperable Lung and Liver Oligometastases from Breast Cancer.**

**Purpose:-** Investigators designed a phase II study to evaluate safety and efficacy of lung and liver stereotactic radiation therapy (SRT) in oligometastatic breast cancer patients unsuitable for surgery, using VMAT RapidArc approach.

**Detailed Description:-** Investigators designed a prospective phase II study to evaluate safety and efficacy of lung and liver stereotactic radiation therapy (SRT) scheduled for oligometastatic breast cancer patients unsuitable for surgery with age major than 18 years old and with adequate performance status (ECOG), using VMAT RapidArc approach.

The potential advantage of this technique is the ability to deliver a more selective irradiation to tumor's target while reducing doses to normal tissue, optimizing the therapeutic window.

**Locations:-** Italy
Istituto Clinico Humanitas - Rozzano, Milano, Italy, 20089.
**Contact:** Fiorenza De Rose, MD +390282247307
fiorenza.de_rose@cancercenter.humanitas.it
**Contact:** Tiziana Comito, MD    +390282247244
tiziana.comito@cancercenter.humanitas.it

## Evaluation of a Novel Infra-red Breast Imaging System for Risk Assessment in Women at High Risk for Breast Cancer.

**Purpose:-** Three-dimensional functional Metabolic Imaging (3D MIRA) is a new infrared imaging technology using the Real Imager 4(RI4) developed by Real Imaging.

This technology generates 3D metabolic maps and based on sophisticated machine learning technology, provides objective risk assessment for the presence of malignant tumor. The procedure is non-invasive, comfortable and does not involve ionizing radiation. Moreover, Real Imaging's 3D Functional MIRA is unaffected by breast density and is therefore ideal for evaluating patients with mammographically dense breasts.

The purpose of this clinical study is to assess the ability of this novel technology to detect clinically occult breast cancer in a cohort of women that are at high risk for breast cancer.

We hypothesize that the combination of screening mammography and metabolic screening (3D MIRA) will result in significantly higher breast cancer detection rates.

**Locations:-**
**Israel:-** The Chaim Sheba Medical Center at Tel-Hashomer
Ramat-Gan, Israel.
**Phone:-** 03-5303295 or 03-5305893
**Email:-** pniot@sheba.health.gov.il

---

## Comparison of the Cosmetic Outcome of Hypofractionated Versus Normofractionated IMRT in Treatment of Breast Cancer (KOSIMA).

**Purpose:-** Several multicenter studies have shown the equivalence of hypofractionated radiotherapy and normofractionated radiotherapy after breast-conserving surgery. However, the treatment in these studies was carried out with conventional techniques and not with the modern IMRT. Also the evaluation of quality of life and cosmetic outcome were not standardized.

This study is a two-arm prospective study comparing normofractionated and hypofractionated radiotherapy in patients with breast cancer using tangential IMRT techniques.

The primary endpoints are acute and chronic cosmetic breast changes. The secondary endpoint is the patients' quality of life.

Patients to be included are breast cancer 60 years old patients or older with tumor stages pTis-pT3, pN0-pN1a, M0 after breast-conserving surgery. Patients with right sided breast cancer are stratified to receive a hypofractionated treatment course (40.05 / 2.67Gy in 15 fractions) and the left sided breast cancer a normofractionated irradiation (50/2Gy in 25 fractions). In both arms, patients between 60-69 years are to receive a boost (16 Gy / 2Gy).

In both groups, a tangential intensity-modulated radiation technique aiming to achieve optimal dose homogeneity is applied.

Since higher single radiation dose to the heart can lead to higher morbidity and/or mortality, patient stratification according to the diseased side was adopted where the left-sided breast cancer patients would receive normofractionated 2Gy single dose. Therefore there is no randomization.

For classification and grading of adverse cosmetic events, the "Common Toxicity Criteria (CTC-AE V3.0) and the recognized LENT-SOMA scores are to be regularly documented. Quality of life is to be documented with two standardized, validated questionnaires "QLQ C30 and BR23" of the EORTC (European Organization for Research and Treatment of Cancer). The questionnaires are to be filled by the patients themselves at different time points during the study period.

A sum of grade III fibrosis, grade III telangiectasia and grade II hyperpigmentation of around 20% is expected after 2 years.

Therefore, calculation of the required number of cases based on an alpha of 0.05 and a power of 80% with a maximal tolerable toxicity difference of 15% within 2 years results in the need for recruiting 226 patients (113 in each arm) (non-inferiority of hypofractionated therapy).

**Locations:-** Germany - Department of Radiotherapy University Hospital Mannheim - Germany, 68167

Theodor-Kutzer-Ufer 1-3 - 68167 Mannheim, Germany.
**Contact:** Frederik Wenz, MD   +496213834960
frederik.wenz@medma.uni-heidelberg.de
**Contact:** Ahmed Yasser Aboumadian, MD      +496213836020
yasser.abomadyan@umm.de

---

## Breast Cancer Toxicity (CANTO).

**Purpose:-** The aims of the cohort will be to quantify impact of cancer treatments toxicities , and to generate predictors of chronic toxicity in patients with non-metastatic breast cancer.
**The project will include four specific aims:-**

1. To develop a database of chronic treatment related toxicity in a cohort of 20 000 women with stage I-III breast cancer (= non metastatic), whatever these treatments are (surgery; radiation therapy; chemotherapy …)
2. To describe incidence, clinical presentation, and outcome of chronic toxicities over a maximum of 8 years.
3. To describe the psychological, the social and the economic impacts of chronic toxicities.
4. To generate predictors for chronic toxicities in order to prevent them, based upon biological criteria.

The expected impact of these toxicities, when identified, will be to improve quality of life and to decrease health cost, by the early identification of patients at high risk of toxicity. Such early identification could lead to prevent toxic effect by: a. developing prevention strategies, b. substituting toxic treatment by a non (less) toxic one.

Also, such cohort will offer a quantification of the impact of treatment toxicity, that could be further used to quantify medical usefulness of strategies that aim at decreasing treatment toxicities (implementation of predictive biomarker for resistance, cytotoxic-free regimen etc).

**Locations:-** France
Gustave roussy - Villejuif, France, 94805
Contact:- Fabrice ANDRE    (0)1 42 11 43 71  ext +33.

**Contact:-** Christel Mesleard    (0)1 44 23 55 51 ext + 33.
c-mesleard@unicancer.fr
Contact:- Anne Laure Martin    (0)1 44 23 55 56
al-martin@unicancer.fr

---

## Evaluation of Effectiveness of Acupuncture on Quality of Life in Patients With Breast Cancer Receiving Chemotherapy.

**Purpose:-** The aim of this trial is to investigate the effectiveness of acupuncture on quality of life in patients with breast cancer receiving chemotherapy compared to routine care.

Inclusion Criteria:

- diagnosed breast cancer (invasive, intraductal, hormone-sensitive and not hormone-sensitive, only locoregional metastases)

- current chemotherapy at Mammazentrum Hamburg with regimen FEC/DOC or EC/DOC
- willingness to receive acupuncture within the next 6 month if randomized in acupuncture group
- willingness to refrain from acupuncture within the next 6 month if randomized in control group
- informed consent

**Locations:-** Germany
Schäferkampsallee 34, Hamburg, Germany - 20357.

**Principal Investigator:-** Martin Carstensen, Prof. MD
Mammazentrum am Krankenhaus Jerusalem, Hamburg, Germany
Tel. 040-44 190-500, Fax 040-44 190-504
info@mammazentrum-hamburg.de

---

**Predictive Clinical and Biological Parameters in Breast Cancer (BC-BIO).**

**Purpose:-** Research of predictive clinical and biological factors in breast cancer: genomic, proteomic, mutation.

**Contact:** Dominique GENRE, MD - 33491223778 -
drci.up@ipc.unicancer.fr
**Contact:** Jihane PAKRADOUNI, PharmD PhD - 33491223778 -
drci.up@ipc.unicancer.fr

**Locations:-** France
Institut Paoli Calmettes
Marseille, France, 13009
Contact: Carole TARPIN, MD     33491223778     drci.up@ipc.unicancer.fr
Principal Investigator: Carole TARPIN, MD
Hôpital Sainte-Musse
Toulon, France
**Contact:** Frédéric VIRET, MD     frederic.viret@ch-toulon.fr

**Anastrozole in Preventing Breast Cancer in Postmenopausal Women at Increased Risk of Breast Cancer (IBIS II).**

**Purpose:-**

**RATIONALE:** Chemoprevention therapy is the use of certain drugs to try to prevent the development of cancer. Anastrozole may be effective in preventing breast cancer.

**PURPOSE:** This randomized clinical trial is studying how well anastrozole works in preventing breast cancer in postmenopausal women who are at increased risk for the disease.

**Locations:-** Queen Mary University of London
Mile End Road
London
E1 4NS

**Contact:-** email: j.cuzick@qmul.ac.uk
Tel: +44 (0) 20 7882 3504

---

**What Matters Most: Choosing the Right Breast Cancer Surgery for You.**

**Purpose:-** What Matters Most is a study that aims to determine how best to help women of lower socioeconomic status make high-quality decisions about early stage breast cancer treatments.

What Matters Most will be comparing two decision aids used in the clinic visit to usual care (what normally happens in the clinic). The first decision aid (Option Grid) presents evidence-based information about lumpectomy and mastectomy in a tabular format using text only.

The second decision aid (Picture Option Grid) presents evidence-based information about lumpectomy and mastectomy using pictures, pictographs and simplified text. What Matters Most aims to show that the interventions can reduce disparities in decision-making and treatment choice between women of high and low SES.

**Locations:-**

United States, Missouri
Washington University in St. Louis
Saint Louis, Missouri, United States, 63110
**Contact:** Mary Politi, PhD
Email:- mpoliti@wustl.edu

United States, New Hampshire
Norris Cotton Cancer Center, Dartmouth-Hitchcock Medical Center
Lebanon, New Hampshire, United States, 03756
**Contact:** Marie-Anne Durand, MSc, PhD
Phone: 603-653-0850
Paige.Stein@dartmouth.edu

United States, New York
Bellevue Hospital Center
New York, New York, United States, 10016
**Contact:** Shubhada Dhage, MD, FACS
Phone:- 212-263-6509
Email:- shubhada.dhage@nyumc.org

NYU Langone Medical Center
New York, New York, United States, 10016
Contact: Shubhada Dhage, MD, FACS
Montefiore Medical Center
The Bronx, New York, United States, 10467
**Contact:** Katie Weichman
Phone: 718-920-4800
Email: aesthetics@montefiore.org

# Triple Negative Breast Cancer: Study of Molecular and Genetic Factors.

**Purpose:-** Breast cancer triples negatives (TN; 15 % of the cases) are characterized by a high histoprognostic grade, a strong proliferation, a strong metastatic power, and a worse prognosis than the other forms of breast cancer.

It is however a heterogenous group for histological and molecular level, but also for evolution. Most of the TN is part of the basal breast cancer subcategory. Until now, the medical treatment is based on chemotherapy.

Breast cancers by constitutional mutation of BRCA1 / BRCA2 (5 % of breast cancers) are mostly of basal type and their prognostic seems better that what could be expected from high grade tumors and without hormonal receptors.

They would be much more frequent in the TN group. However, at this day, no prospective study was led to estimate this incidence, or to study the intervention of other genes of predisposition, as well to analyze the links between this phenotype and their consequences at the germinal or somatic level, in terms of associated molecular changes and prognosis.

The purpose of this study is, on a prospective study, to lead a joined analysis at the germinal level, in search of mutations of the main genes of breast cancer predisposition (BRCA1/2, PALB2, PTEN, PALB2), and at the tumor level (tissue micro-array and transcriptome), by correlating these results to the main clinical parameters.

The 5 years relapse-free survival will also be estimated.

Locations:- France
Centre jean Perrin
Clermont-Ferrand, France, 63011
Hospital La Timone

Marseille, France, 13005

Institut Paoli-Calmettes
Marseille, France, 13009

Centre Antoine Lacassagne
Nice, France, 06189

**Principal Investigator:-** Jean-Marc EXTRA, MD
Institute Paoli-Calmettes
**Telephone:-** 33-0-4-91-22-35-37
**E-mail:-** extrajm@marseille.fnclcc.fr

**Know Your Risk: Assessment at Screening for Breast Cancer - Pilot Study (KYRAS).**

**Purpose:-** The purpose of this pilot study is to evaluate a decision support website (RealRisks) designed to inform patients about breast cancer chemoprevention. It is coupled with a physician-centered (BNAV) decision support website as part of clinical workflow in the primary care setting.

The investigator hypothesizes that improving accuracy of breast cancer risk perception and understanding of the risks/benefits of chemoprevention will enhance informed decision-making and uptake of breast cancer prevention strategies in the primary care setting.

**Detailed Description:-** Breast cancer is the most common malignancy among women in the U.S. and the primary prevention of this disease is a major public health issue.

The U.S. Preventive Services Task Force and other professional organizations recommend that clinicians discuss chemoprevention with high-risk women. Breast cancer chemoprevention with anti-estrogens, such as tamoxifen, raloxifene, exemestane, and anastrozole, is under-

utilized, despite several randomized controlled trials demonstrating a 40 65% decrease in breast cancer incidence among high-risk women.

Compounding this underutilization is the fact that a large proportion of women may be unaware of their high-risk status due to the investigators inability to adequately screen them in the primary care setting.

Further research is needed to determine how knowledge about breast cancer, actual/perceived risk, and risks/benefits of chemoprevention are best communicated to women in order to promote breast cancer prevention strategies.

This study assesses risk communication and shared decision-making in patient-clinician dyads by administering validated measures at baseline, after interacting with the tools prior to the clinic visit, and after the clinical visit (quantitative analysis); and by using observer-based methods of audio-tape recordings of their clinical encounters (qualitative analysis).

The investigator hypothesizes that combining a patient-centered decision aid with a physician-centered decision support tool integrated into clinic workflow will improve accuracy of breast cancer risk perception, facilitate referrals for specialized risk counseling, and increase chemoprevention uptake.

**Locations:-** United States, New York
Columbia University Medical Center
New York, New York, United States, 10032

**Principal Investigator:-** Katherine D Crew, M.D., M.S.
**Tel:-** 212-305-5098
**e-mail:-** kd59@columbia.edu

## Cryoablation of Low Risk Small Breast Cancer- Ice3 Trial.

**Purpose:-** To evaluate the efficacy of cryoablation without lumpectomy and its impact on local and distant recurrence of early stage breast cancer.

**Locations:-** United States, California

BreastLink
Santa Ana, California, United States, 92705
Principal Investigator: Lisa Curcio, MD

United States, Connecticut
Bridgeport Hospital, Yale Medical School
Trumbull, Connecticut, United States, 06611
Principal Investigator: Andrew Kenler, MD

United States, Georgia
Dalton Surgical Group
Dalton, Georgia, United States, 30720
Principal Investigator: Eric R Manahan, MD

United States, Indiana
Indiana University
Indianapolis, Indiana, United States, 46202-5116
Principal Investigator: Linda K Han, MD

United States, Michigan
Karmanos Cancer Institute
Detroit, Michigan, United States, 48201
Principal Investigator: Hussein D Aoun, MD

Regional Medical Imaging
Flint, Michigan, United States, 48507

Principal Investigator: Randy Hicks, MD
Comprehensive Breast Care

Troy, Michigan, United States, 48085
Principal Investigator: Linsey Gold, MD

United States, New Jersey
CentraState Medical Center
Freehold, New Jersey, United States, 07728
Principal Investigator: Kenneth Tomkovich, MD

United States, New Mexico
Breast Specialty care
Albuquerque, New Mexico, United States, 87114
Sub-Investigator: Susan Seedman
United States, New York
Mount Sinai Beth Israel
New York, New York, United States, 10011
Principal Investigator: Sarah Cate, MD

Columbia University/ NY Presbyterian hospital
New York, New York, United States, 10032
Principal Investigator: Sheldon Feldman
Weill Cornell Medical College
New York, New York, United States, 10065
Principal Investigator: Rache Simmons, MD

United States, Ohio
Cincinnati Breast Surgeons Inc.
Cincinnati, Ohio, United States, 45227
Principal Investigator: Karen S Columbus, MD

United States, Pennsylvania
Thomas Jefferson University hospital
Philadelphia, Pennsylvania, United States, 19107
Principal Investigator: Alexander Sevrukov, MD

United States, Tennessee

West Clinic
Germantown, Tennessee, United States, 38138
Principal Investigator: Richard E. Fine, MD

United States, Texas
Complete Breast Care
Plano, Texas, United States, 75075
Principal Investigator: Beth Anglin, MD

United States, Wisconsin
Wheaton Franciscan Medical Group- Comprehensive breast care
Franklin, Wisconsin, United States, 53132
Principal Investigator: Jodi L Brehm, MD

**Contact:-** Elisabeth Sadka
+972-4-6230333 ext 223
**Email:-** elisabeth@icecure-medical.com

## To Enhance Breast Cancer Survivorship of Asian Americans (TICAA).

**Purpose:-** The purpose of the proposed randomized intervention study is to test the efficacy of the technology-based information and coaching/support program for Asian American breast cancer survivors (TICAA) in enhancing the women's breast cancer survivorship experience at three time points (pre-test, post1-month, and post 3-month).

**Detailed Description:-** Despite few studies on Asian American breast cancer survivors, it is well known that these women shoulder unnecessary burden of breast cancer because they rarely complain about symptoms or pain, delay seeking help, and rarely ask or get support due to their cultural values and beliefs and language barriers.

This demonstrates a definite need for support in this specific population. However, survivorship programs that are increasingly instituted at cancer centers have serious impediments to providing information and coaching/support because of the lack of staff time and insurance reimbursement. Furthermore, the pressure of fast-paced clinical patient-provider interactions leaves little time for health care providers to provide up-to-date information and coaching or support for these women based on their cultural attitudes.

All these circumstances necessitate an innovative and creative delivery method of information and coaching/support. A technology- based approach using computers and mobile devices (smart phones and tablets) promises to meet this necessity with high flexibility and accessibility, and minimizes the cost of the intervention in busy and costly health care settings.

Also, a technology-based intervention that does not involve face-to-face interactions could work better for many women from cultures where breast cancer is still a stigmatizing experience.

Therefore, based on Preliminary Studies (PSs), the research team has developed and pilot-tested a theory-driven technology-based information and coaching/support program that is culturally tailored to Asian American breast cancer survivors using multiple features.

The purpose of the proposed randomized intervention study is to test the efficacy of the technology-based information and coaching/support program for Asian American breast cancer survivors (TICAA) in enhancing the women's breast cancer survivorship experience.

The specific aims are to: a) determine whether the intervention group will show significantly greater improvements than the control group in primary outcomes (needs for help, physical and psychological symptoms, and quality of life) from baseline (pre-test) to Time Points 1 (post 1-month) and 2 (post 3-months); b) identify theory-based variables (attitudes, self-efficacy, perceived barriers, and social influences related to breast cancer survivorship) that mediate the intervention effects of the TICAA on the primary outcomes at the three time points (pre-test, post 1-month and post 3-months); and c) determine whether the effects of the

TICAA on the primary outcomes are moderated by background characteristics and disease factors. The proposed study will be guided by the Bandura's Theory of Behavioral Change.

This study adopts a randomized repeated measures pretest/posttest control group design in 330 Asian American breast cancer survivors. The long-term goals are to: (a) implement the program into various health care settings; (b) determine if the TICAA will lead to long-term improved health outcomes; and (c) fundamentally enhance the methodology/paradigm of culturally tailored technology-based interventions for ethnic minority groups of breast cancer survivors.

**Locations:-** United States, North Carolina
Duke University, School of Nursing
Durham, North Carolina, United States, 27710
**Contact:-** Eun-Ok Im, PhD, MPH
**Tel:-** 919-668-3838
**Email:-** eun-ok.im@duke.edu

---

## Evaluating Anti-PD-L1 Antibody (Durvalumab) Plus Anti-CTLA-4 Antibody (Tremelimumab) in HR+/HER2- Breast Cancer.

**Purpose:-** The goal of this clinical research study is to find the highest dose combination of tremelimumab and durvalumab [also called MEDI4736]) that can be given before standard of care pre-surgery chemotherapy to patients with HR+, HER2- breast cancer.

Researchers also want to learn more about how certain immune cells may change in the body when they are given the drug combination. Researchers also want to find out how patients with HR+, HER2- breast cancer respond to the study drugs before they receive standard chemotherapy treatment.

**Locations:-** United States, Texas

University of Texas MD Anderson Cancer Center
Houston, Texas, United States, 77030

**Contact:-** Elizabeth A. Mittendorf, MD, PHD
Tel:-713-745-2840
**Email:-** CR_Study_Registration@mdanderson.org

---

## Genotyping 2 SNPs in Chinese Breast Cancers.

**Purpose:-** The purpose of this study is to determine the frequency of two Single Nucleotide Polymorphisms (SNPs) by sanger-sequencing in Breast Cancers and healthy controls.

**Detailed Description:** Since the 1990s breast cancers incidence of china has increased more than twice as fast as global rates. Chinese patients are responsible for 12.2% of all newly diagnosed breast cancers and 9.6% of all deaths to world breast cancers.

Breast cancer is now the second frequently diagnosed cancer and is the leading cause of cancer-related death in Chinese women.

Two of the most prevalent breast cancer susceptibility genes are BRCA1and BRCA2. However, because of population based Genetic heterogeneity, the frequency of BRCA1/BRCA2 mutation is not as high in Caucasian population as in China.

Anyway, the mean age at diagnosis of breast cancer in China is almost 10 years younger and more cases are diagnosed before 40 than those in Caucasians. Therefore, it is believed that there are certain specific susceptibility loci in Chinese breast cancers.

In preliminary experiments, investigators found two germline mutations may associate with Chinese breast cancers.
The purpose of the study is to determine the frequency of two germline

mutations by sanger-sequencing in a larger sample of Chinese breast cancers.

**Locations:-** China, Shaanxi
The First Affiliated Hospital of Fourth Military Medical University
Xi'an, Shaanxi, China, 710000

**Contact:** Hongping Song, Ph.D
**Tel:-** +86-29-84771663
**Email:-** Songhp@fmmu.edu.cn

---

## Breast MRI in Women With Known or Suspected Breast Cancer and in Healthy Participants.

### Purpose:-

**RATIONALE:-** Diagnostic procedures, such as MRI, may help diagnose breast cancer. It may also help doctors predict a patient's response to treatment.

**PURPOSE:-** This clinical trial is studying breast MRI in women with known or suspected breast cancer and in healthy participants.

### Primary Outcome Measures:-

Feasibility of advanced, quantitative, multi-parametric magnetic resonance imaging (MRI) methods for characterizing breast tumors to develop potential surrogate imaging markers for diagnosis and prediction of treatment response [Time Frame: on-study date and at 6 months, up to 4 years]

Quantitative, multi-parametric MRI imaging methods include Dynamic Contrast MRI, Diffusion Weighted MRI, and Magnetic Resonance Spectroscopy. Patients will include healthy female volunteers and women diagnosed with breast cancer. Time frames begin at study entry (healthy volunteers), pre-surgical and pre- and post-chemotherapy (breast cancer patients).

**Locations:-** United States, Tennessee
Vanderbilt-Ingram Cancer Center
Nashville, Tennessee, United States, 37232-6838

**Principal Investigator:** Bapsi Chak, MD
**Email:-** bapsi.chak@vanderbilt.edu
**Tel:-** 800-811-8480
615-322-2555
**Physicians:** 1-877-936-8422

---

## 99mTc-3PRGD2 SPECT/CT in Breast Cancer Patients.

**Purpose:-**This is an open-label SPECT/CT (single photon emission computed tomography / computed tomography) study to investigate clinical study of 99mTc-3PRGD2 SPECT/CT in diagnosis and efficacy evaluation of breast cancer. Diagnostic group: for patients in suspicion of breast cancer.

The standard of truth for diagnosis was based on histopathologic findings after surgical removal of the tumor or a definite diagnosis from fine needle aspiration biopsy. A single dose of nearly 0.3 mCi/kg (milli-Curie/kilogram) body weight of 99mTc-3PRGD2 ( ≤ 20 µg 3PRGD2) will be intravenously injected into the patients. Visual and semiquantitative method will be used to assess the whole-body planar and lesions SPECT/CT images.

Efficacy evaluation group: for patients firstly diagnose with malignant tumors (breast cancer), and prepare to chemotherapy(including neoadjuvant chemotherapy) or radiotherapy.
The standard of truth for diagnosis was based on histopathologic findings

after fine needle aspiration biopsy. A single dose of nearly 0.3 mCi/kg body weight of 99mTc-3PRGD2 (≤ 20 μg 3PRGD2) will be intravenously injected into the patients before treatment, the second period, sixth period.

Visual, semiquantitative method will be used to assess the whole-body planar and lesions SPECT/CT images. By comparing with result of the other related imaging, for instance, PET/CT (positron emission tomography/computed tomography), CT (computed tomography), MRI (magnetic resonance imaging), Doppler Ultrasound, Mammography, etc.

**Locations:-** China, Fujian
Department of Nuclear Medicine, First Affiliated Hospital of Fujian Medical University
Fuzhou, Fujian, China, 350005

**Contact:-** Weibing Miao, MD   +86 591 87981618
**Email:-** miaoweibing@126.com

**Contact:-** Zhenying Chen, MB   +86 591 87981619
**Email:-** 714144972@qq.com

---

## Metastatic Breast Cancer Treatment Planning.

**Purpose:-** The overarching objective of this study is to close clinical knowledge and performance gaps by providing oncology clinicians with the latest advances and emerging research in the evidence-based and personalized treatment of metastatic breast cancer patients.

In addition, the research team seeks to meet quality measures relevant to value-based care delivery through IT infrastructure and clinical workflow processes.

The research team also hopes to gain insights into clinician practice patterns related to metastatic breast cancer, and the correlation between the reported goals of care for patients with metastatic breast cancer, and the patients' fit/frailty status and treatment decisions.

**Contact:-** Laura DiGiovanni
**Tel:-** 800-460-3790
**Email:-** laura@carevive.com

---

## Assessing Impact of Loco-regional Treatment on Survival in Metastatic Breast Cancer at Presentation.

**Purpose:-** Traditionally metastatic breast cancer patients are not offered loco-regional treatment except in cases of fungation or bleeding. However, scientific evidence for such omission of loco-regional treatment in metastatic breast cancer patients is lacking.

On one hand, studies have shown that removal of primary tumor at times leads to complete disappearance of metastases and improvement in survival in renal cell carcinoma patients.

However, such studies have never been performed in other solid tumors. On the other hand, there is a strong body of evidence in experimental settings that show that removal of primary tumor allows growth of metastasis.

There is lack of similar data in humans in clinical settings. Offering loco-regional treatment in metastatic breast cancer patients in a setting of randomized controlled trial will help in improving survival of such patients and understanding the natural history of breast cancer.

**Locations:-** India
Tata Memorial Hospital
Mumbai, Maharashtra, India, 400 012

**Principal Investigator:-** Rajendra A Badwe, MS (Surgery).
**E-mail:** badwera@tmc.gov.in
**Tel:-** +91-22-24139318

---

**Study of Radiation Exposure and Bilateral Breast Cancer.**

**Purpose:-** This study is being done to find out what factors may be related to the risk of getting a second breast cancer among women who already have breast cancer in one breast. It will look at how genes, treatment for breast cancer; including radiation therapy, and the effects of different lifestyle activities, may affect the risk of breast cancer.

It will use different processes to find genes that might increase the risk of breast cancer. The results of this study may help to develop better ways to detect, treat and prevent breast cancer. This study will compare women who have breast cancer in both breasts to women who have breast cancer in only one breast.

**Locations:-** United States, California

Cancer Prevention Institute of California
Fremont, California, United States, 94538

United States, Iowa
University of Iowa
Iowa City, Iowa, United States, 52242

United States, New York
Memorial Sloan Kettering Cancer Center
New York, New York, United States, 10065

United States, Washington
Fred Hutchinson Cancer Research Center
Seattle, Washington, United States, 98109

Canada
Ontario Cancer Registry-Fu Study
Ontario, Canada

**Principal Investigator:-** Jonine Bernstein, PhD
Memorial Sloan Kettering Cancer Center

**Tel:-** 646-888-8241
**Email:-** bernstej@mskcc.org

---

## Cyclophosphamide and Vaccine Therapy With or Without Trastuzumab in Treating Patients With Metastatic Breast Cancer.

### Purpose:-

**RATIONALE:-** Vaccines made from gene-modified tumor cells may help the body build an effective immune response to kill tumor cells. Biological therapies, such as cyclophosphamide and trastuzumab, may increase the number of immune cells and make the immune response stronger.

It is not yet known whether giving cyclophosphamide together with vaccine therapy is more effective with or without trastuzumab in treating patients with metastatic breast cancer.

**PURPOSE:-** This randomized phase II trial is studying the side effects of giving cyclophosphamide together with vaccine therapy and to see how well it works compared with giving cyclophosphamide and vaccine therapy together with trastuzumab in treating patients with metastatic breast cancer.

**Locations:-** United States, Maryland
Sidney Kimmel Comprehensive Cancer Center at Johns Hopkins
Baltimore, Maryland, United States, 21231-2410

**Principal Investigator:-** Leisha A. Emens, MD, PhD
**Tel:-** 410-502-7051
**Email:-** emensle@jhmi.edu

---

**Chimeric Antigen Receptor-Modified T Cells for Breast Cancer.**

**Purpose:-** The purpose of this study is to evaluate the safety and efficacy of HER2-CAR-T cell Infusion for advanced HER2 positive breast cancer.

**Locations:-** China, Guangdong
Central laboratory in Fuda Cancer Hospital
Guangzhou, Guangdong, China, 510000

**Contact:-** Jibing Chen, PhD
**Tel:-** +86-18903068207
**Email:-** jibingchen398@163.com

Central laboratory in Fuda Cancer Hospital
Guangzhou, Guangdong, China, 510000
**Contact:-** Huimin Tao, PhD
**Tel:-** +86-18927563958
**Email:-** 747064551@qq.com

---

**Attention and Interpretation Modification (AIM) for Fear of Breast Cancer Recurrence: An Intervention Development Study.**

**Purpose:-** The purpose of this study is to customize and personalize an existing computer-based intervention program in order to help breast cancer survivors cope with fears of cancer recurrence.

**Locations:-** United States, New York
Memorial Sloan-Kettering Cancer Center

New York, New York, United States, 10065

**Principal Investigator:-** Wendy Lichtenthal, PhD
**Phone:-** 646-888-4812
**Email:-** lichtenw@mskcc.org

---

**Medico-economic Study of Three Strategies of Sentinel Lymph Node Analysis in Operable Breast Cancer (SAGE).**

**Purpose:-** Breast carcinoma requires frequently an adjuvant therapy after surgical excision: in this way, one of the major criteria indicating the need of adjuvant chemotherapy is the diagnosis of a metastatic lymph-node invasion, mainly in the axillary field.

Axillary surgery is therefore mandatory at the diagnosis of breast carcinoma. For many years, in order to avoid unnecessary complications due to extensive axillary surgery (for instance, arm enlargement by lymphedema), a limited surgery is frequently performed on the first supposed invaded lymph-nodes (LN) called "sentinel" LN technique; if the sentinel LN are not invaded, extensive axillary surgery can be omitted.

To decide it during the surgery, removed sentinel LN are cut in 3 to 4 slices which are examined immediately as smears (cytology) or frozen slices (pathology). However, due to hazard in cutting the LN, micro-metastases can be misdiagnosed.

That is why a recent molecular biology method has been developed in which the total LN are crushed and blended, then analyzed by OSNA technique (One Step Nuclear Acid analysis) so as to amplify and detect the mRNA coding for cytokeratin-19 protein witnessing the LN metastatic invasion. A standardized automated technique is available with a mean time of 30 to 50 minutes according to the number of analyzed LN.

In 12 international studies (2830 cases) the consistency between OSNA technique and final pathology is of 91 to 98% and the sensitivity seems higher. Less than 5% of all breast carcinomas cells don't express CK-19 protein.

The use of OSNA technique requires a dedicated machine and a skilled pathologist, increasing slightly the operation time; however it allows to avoid the immediate and long-term complications due to the radical LN axillary surgery in case of negativity of the sentinel LN procedure.

To date, the three techniques including extemporaneous examinations (OSNA or classical methods) or not (classical pathological analysis) have their own advantages and drawbacks.

"SAGE" study main objective is to compare these three techniques in terms of direct costs and Quality of Life impacts. The superiority of any of these three techniques is not the purpose of SAGE study, but the economic burden of OSNA technique in comparison with the 2 others in the standard setting in France.

Quality of Life and Pain evaluations will be performed immediately after surgery and during the 6 months after.

**Locations:-** France
ICO Paul Papin
Angers, France, 49000
**Contact:-** Pedro RARO, MD
**Email:-** pedro.raro@ico.unicancer.fr

Principal Investigator: Pedro RARO, Md
ICO René Gauducheau
Nantes - St Herblain, France, 44800
**Contact:-** Virginie BORDES, MD
**Tel:-** +33 2 40 67 99 00 ext 9185
**Email:-** Virginie.Bordes@ico.unicancer.fr
**Principal Investigator:-** Virginie BORDES, MD

Institut Curie
Paris, France, 75248
**Contact:-** Séverine ALRAN, MD
**Email:-** severine.alran@curie.net
**Principal Investigator:-** Séverine ALRAN, MD

## Homeopathic Protocol for Advanced Breast Cancer.

**Purpose:-** The objective of this study is to conduct a feasibility study at Meir Oncology Institute examining whether patients with advanced breast cancer would follow a homeopathic protocol for three to six months.

The primary aim of the study is to establish if patients with advanced breast cancer in Meir Oncology Institute would follow a regimen of treatment as used by Dr Banerji in India, for six months.

The secondary aim is to observe the quality of life and wellbeing of patients undergoing this protocol.

### Detailed Description:-

- Homeopathy is a controversial system of care and at the center of the controversy lays the question of whether high dilution remedies can be effective.

There have been only a handful of high quality studies of homeopathy on the treatment of cancer, despite its widespread use for this condition.

In a recent prospective observational study done in Germany with cancer patients in two differently treated cohorts it was observed that an improvement in quality of life was observed in patients taking the addition of homeopathic treatment.

In the laboratory, research on homeopathy and cancer that does exist is limited but has some clues for effects that cannot be ignored.

A study that was conducted at The University of Texas MD Anderson Cancer Center, revealed that four ultradilute remedies (Carcinosin, Phytolacca, Conium, and Thuja) exerted preferential cytotoxic effects against two breast cancer cell lines, causing cell cycle delay/arrest and apoptosis without affecting the normal mammary epithelial cells.

Since patients with advanced breast cancer are the highest CAM users amongst patients affected by cancer, it was thought that a feasibility study with this group of patients, would be a rational first step in proceeding to evaluate this controversial method of care, if it has merit or not.

- The objective of this study is to conduct a feasibility study at Meir Oncology Institute examining whether patients with advanced breast cancer would follow a homeopathic protocol for three to six months. The primary aim of the study is to establish if patients with advanced breast cancer in Meir Oncology Institute would follow homeopathic protocol as used by Dr Banerji in India, for six months. The secondary aim is to observe the quality of life and wellbeing of patients undergoing this protocol.
- Patients with the diagnosis of advanced breast cancer who attend the Meir Oncology Institute clinic will be offered by their treating physician or nurse a fact sheet about this study and will be asked to participate in this protocol. The protocol will be explained to the patient by the research team. If they agree to participate they will be given a consent form to sign, and basic information will be obtained from each patient. This information will include basic demographics (age, marital status, employment, education level) and basic medical information (Disease status and progress, current symptoms, medications and treatments being used, complementary medicine being used) as well as evaluation of quality of life using the European Organization for Research and Treatment of Cancer (EORTC) quality of life questionnaire (QLQ).

- Patients will receive the selected homeopathic remedies (Carcinosin 30C, Phytolacca 200C, and Thuja 30C) with written instructions about the proper use of the remedies. The remedies will be offered to patients in addition to their regular conventional care. Patients that cannot participate in conventional cancer care due to side-effects, expected adverse reactions or other reasons that prevent them from utilizing conventional care will be offered to participate in the study, as well.
- In addition, patients who for their own reasons elect to refuse conventional treatment can be offered to participate in the study in order to keep them in the system and not lose them to alternative untested treatments.
- Every 4 weeks for the period of 3 months and once at 6 months, a research assistant/ research nurse will contact each participant to review EORTC QLQ- C-30 questionnaire to evaluate quality of life as well as a follow up questionnaire which will verify the actual use of these remedies, perceived problems in taking these remedies, utilization of other therapies, address patients concerns, and document disease progression.
- A total of 30 patients will be enrolled in this study and their data will be reviewed and analyzed six months after recruitment to the study.

**Locations:-** Israel
Institute of Oncology Meir Medical Center
Kfar Saba, Israel
**Principal Investigator:-** Moshe Frenkel, MD
**Email:-** frenkelm@netvision.net.il
**Tel:-** 02-5665476 or 052-8313914

---

**Magnetic Resonance Imaging of the Whole Body, Including Diffusion, in the Medical Evaluation of Breast Cancers at High Risk for Metastasis and the Follow-up of Metastatic Cancers.**

**Purpose:-** Whole-body MRI including diffusion is a booming technique. Numerous studies have demonstrated its interest in metastatic cancers. Breast cancers, especially hormone-sensitive ones, are very osteophilic and bones are the most frequent metastatic site.

Apart from morphological criteria (lesion size and RECIST criteria), MRI provides quantitative functional criteria (diffusion and ADC values).

According to a recent study, whole body MRI is as good as PET/CT and more effective than bone scintigraphy for the diagnosis of bone metastases for cancers of breast and prostate with a high metastatic risk.

Therefore, it seems appropriate to study the performance of whole body MRI in the pre-therapeutic assessment of breast cancer with a high risk for metastasis and the monitoring of metastatic breast cancer.

**Detailed Description:-** Whole-body MRI including diffusion is a booming technique. Numerous studies have demonstrated its interest in metastatic cancers.

Breast cancers, especially hormone-sensitive ones, are very osteophilic and bones are the most frequent metastatic site. Other sites include the lungs, liver, pleura, distant lymph nodes, soft tissue and the central nervous system.

Metastasis are located exclusively in the bones in 30% of the cases. The most commonly affected bones include the axial skeleton, rich in hematopoietic bone marrow : column, pelvis, skull, ribs, clavicles, the proximal part of the femur and humerus.

Five percent of breast cancers are directly metastatic and 20 to 30% of localized breast cancers progress to metastatic stage. This potentially affects a large number of patients, with a median survival of 30 to 36 months.Patients with bone metastases only have a better survival rate than others: 20% at 5 years. It is therefore important to use a reliable and reproducible examination for the monitoring of treatment response.

Apart from morphological criteria (lesion size and RECIST criteria), MRI provides quantitative functional criteria (diffusion and ADC values).

According to a recent study, whole body MRI is as good as PET/CT and more effective than bone scintigraphy for the diagnosis of bone metastases for cancers of breast and prostate with a high metastatic risk. However, this is a preliminary study with a limited and heterogeneous cohort of patients.

Therefore, it seems appropriate to study the performance of whole body MRI in the pre-therapeutic assessment of breast cancer with a high risk for metastasis and the monitoring of metastatic breast cancer.

**Locations:-** Belgium
CHU Brugmann
Brussels, Belgium, 1020
**Principal Investigator:-** Nathalie Hottat, MD
**Tel:-** 003224772434
**Email:-** Nathalie.HOTTAT@chu-brugmann.be

---

## Monitoring Plasma Tumor DNA in Early-Stage Breast Cancer.

**Purpose:-** This study is being done to see if it is possible to use blood samples to predict response to treatment in breast cancer patients receiving preoperative (or neoadjuvant) therapy. Research has shown that most breast cancers release tumor-specific DNA into the blood (that is, DNA that is specific to the tumor cells or cancer).

This DNA can be detected in blood testing known as plasma tumor-DNA or "ptDNA."

This DNA is separate from that found in the blood and tissue samples which serve as the "instruction book" or "genetic code" for the cells that make-up the human body.

The changes in ptDNA before and after treatment, as well as after surgery, may also help investigators to understand more about a patient's risk of cancer returning and long-term outcomes.

**Detailed Description:-** This is a prospectively designed study. Up to 229 newly diagnosed invasive HER2-positive or triple-negative breast cancer patients planning neoadjuvant therapy (NAT) will be enrolled.

Blood samples will be collected pre-operatively at the time of diagnosis/prior to NAT, post-cycle 1/pre-cycle 2 of NAT, after all NAT/immediately before surgery, and post-operatively at 6, 12, 24, and 36 months, and annually thereafter if funding allows.

Researchers will also collect representative tissue samples from the diagnostic biopsy (in all participants) and definitive surgery (if available). Additionally, to look at feasibility of tumor DNA analyses in urine samples, urine samples will be collected along with blood samples (urine tumor DNA or utDNA).

Next generation sequencing will be performed on core biopsies of all enrolled patients for tumor-specific mutations (TSM) discovery. Based on those findings, droplet digital PCR (ddPCR) on plasma DNA samples will also be performed to confirm the presence of the TSM in the plasma on diagnosis, and one TSM will be chosen to track as the plasma tumor DNA (ptDNA) mutation of interest.

Investigators will perform ddPCR on pre-operative plasma DNA samples and will assess for the presence of ptDNA. Pathologists will assess surgical specimens for pathologic response (such as complete response/pCR and residual cancer burden/RCB).

As primary endpoint, investigators will assess the number of patients with and without preoperative ptDNA who have pCR versus residual disease.

As exploratory endpoints, the following will also be performed: (a) quantitative multiplex methylation-specific PCR (QM-MSP) in diagnostic biopsy and definitive residual surgery specimen; and, (b) the circulating methylated tumor DNA (cMethDNA) assay in plasma specimens (baseline and after NAT), and evaluate associations with pathologic response.

Additional endpoints include the association between plasma and tissue markers at baseline, after NAT, and (if available) during surveillance with long-term prognosis (invasive disease-free survival/IDFS and distant disease-free survival/DDFS).

**Locations:-** United States, Maryland
Sidney Kimmel Comprehensive Cancer Center at Johns Hopkins
Baltimore, Maryland, United States, 21287

**Principal Investigator:-** Ben Ho Park, M.D., Ph.D.
**Tel:-** 410-955-8804
**Email:-** HopkinsBreastTrials@jhmi.edu

---

**Comparison of CNB and Surgical Specimens for ER, PgR, HER2 Status and Ki67 Index in Invasive Breast Cancer.**

**Purpose:-** This is a prospective, single-center, non-randomized, non-controlled study.

The estrogen receptor (ER), progesterone receptor (PgR), HER2 status and Ki67 index of CNB specimen are critical biomarkers for making neoadjuvant therapy strategy in invasive breast cancer. The concordance of these biomarkers between CNB and surgical specimen was varied in previous retrospective reports. The aim of this study is to determine the discordance of these biomarkers between CNB and surgical specimen and the influence of making treatment strategy by the discordance.

**Locations:-** China, Beijing
Peking University Cancer Hospital
Beijing, Beijing, China, 100142
**Contact:** Zhao-Qing Fan, MD
Tel:-861068236666 ext 8018

---

## Ritonavir and Its Effects on Biomarkers in Women Undergoing Surgery for Newly Diagnosed Breast Cancer.

**Purpose:-** RATIONALE: Ritonavir may stop the growth of tumor cells by blocking some of the enzymes needed for cancer cell growth. Studying samples of blood and tissue from patients with breast cancer in the laboratory may help doctors learn more about the effects of ritonavir on biomarkers involved in breast cancer growth.

**PURPOSE:-** This phase I/II trial is studying the best dose of ritonavir and its effects on biomarkers in women undergoing surgery for newly diagnosed breast cancer.

**Locations:-** United States, Minnesota
Masonic Cancer Center, University of Minnesota
Minneapolis, Minnesota, United States, 55455

United States, Pennsylvania
The Kimmel Cancer Center at Jefferson University
Philadelphia, Pennsylvania, United States, 19107

**Principal Investigator:-** David A. Potter, M.D., Ph.D.
**Tel:-** 612-625-8933 office
**Tel:-** 612-626-7207 lab
**E-mail:-** dapotter@umn.edu

**Comparative Study on Two Post-operative Adjuvant Chemotherapy Regimens for Treating Triple-negative Breast Cancer.**

**Purpose:-** Recent clinical studies showed that triple-negative breast cancer patients (ER-/PR-/HER2-) may benefit more from Capecitabine chemotherapy. However, the optimum post-operative adjuvant Capecitabine chemotherapy regimen has not been determined for Chinese population with triple-negative breast cancer. Thus it's necessary to conduct a multi-center Phase III clinical trial to verify efficacy and safety of Capecitabine in the treatment of triple-negative breast cancer.

In this study, a prospective, randomized, open, multi-center Phase III clinical study was conducted to compare efficacy and safety of sequential Docetaxel followed by Fluorouracil/Epirubicin/Cyclophosphamide (FEC) and sequential Docetaxel and Capecitabine followed by Capecitabine/Epirubicin/Cyclophosphamide (XEC) as post-operative adjuvant chemotherapy in the treatment of triple-negative breast cancer in Chinese population.

**Primary Outcome Measures:-** 5-year disease free survival [Time Frame: 5 year after the completion of chemotherapy]

Including local relapse, distant metastasis, contralateral breast cancer, second primary cancer or death from any cause

**Detailed Description:-** Post-operative adjuvant chemotherapy has been shown to improve overall survival, delay local relapse and reduce distant metastasis by multiple large-scale prospective clinical trial. In registry clinical trial for Capecitabine conducted by O Shaughnessy, it revealed that a combined chemotherapy of Capecitabine and Docetaxel achieved better outcomes compared with Docetaxel alone.
And the significant effect of Capecitabine was also evidenced by CHAT trial in which Trastuzumab/Docetaxel/Capecitabine regimen was proved to perform greater than Trastuzumab/Docetaxel regimen.

In addition to better outcomes, Capecitabine also showed good tolerance and safety profile.

In 2009, Finnish Breast Cancer Group published their study results from FinXX clinical trial on Lancet Oncology, and in this trial, they compared the efficacy between sequential Docetaxel (3 cycles) followed by 3 cycles of Fluorouracil/Epirubicin/Cyclophosphamide (FEC) and sequential Docetaxel and Capecitabine (3 cycles) followed by 3 cycles of Capecitabine/Epirubicin/Cyclophosphamide (XEC) in lymph positive or high-risk lymph negative early-stage breast cancer patients.

And their results showed a better outcome in TX-XEC regimen. 5-year follow-up analysis of this trial revealed that combined Capecitabine regimen can bring more significant clinical benefits to triple-negative breast cancer patients.

Another clinical trial NO1062 released their preliminary results on comparison of AC-T and AC-XT regimens and it showed that combined Capecitabine regimen can significantly improve overall survival and this effect is more obvious in triple--negative breast cancer patients.

Based on the results of FinXX and NO1062, it's of great value to optimize combined Capecitabine regimen and clarify involved questions, such as whether the efficacy of Capecitabine is related to its treatment course or not, whether Capecitabine should be combined into current standardized chemotherapy or a sequential therapy.

Also, there are still no clear conclusions on the best post-operative adjuvant chemotherapy for triple--negative breast cancer patients.

Especially in Chinese population, the efficacy and safety of Capecitabine in adjuvant chemotherapy has not been well established. So it's necessary to explore reasonable dosage, safety profile and efficacy of combined Capecitabine therapy. Based on this purpose, this study is hoped to compare efficacy and safety of sequential Docetaxel followed by

Fluorouracil/Epirubicin/Cyclophosphamide (FEC) and sequential Docetaxel and Capecitabine followed by Capecitabine/Epirubicin/Cyclophosphamide (XEC) as post-operative adjuvant chemotherapy in the treatment of triple-negative breast cancer in Chinese population.

**Location:-** China
Fudan University Shanghai Cancer Center, Shanghai, Shanghai 200032, China.
**Principal Investigator:-** Zhimin Shao, M.D.
**Tel:-** 86-21-54237900
**Email:-** zhimingshao@yahoo.com

## Longitudinal Evaluation of Taxane Induced Neuropathy in Early Stage Breast Cancer.

**Purpose:-** Longitudinal Evaluation of Taxane induced neuropathy in early stage breast cancer.

**Locations:-** United States, Ohio
Ohio State University Wexner Medical Center
Columbus, Ohio, United States, 43210

**Principal Investigator:-** Maryam Lustberg, MD, MPH
**Tel:-** 614-293-8858
**Email:-** Maryam.lustberg@osumc.edu

## Multicenter Phase II Study of Apatinib in Patients With Advanced

**Breast Cancer.**

**Purpose:-** The treatment of the patients with recurrent and metastatic breast cancer remains a major problem. There is still a lack of effective targeted therapy for Her-2 negative breast cancer.

Based on the present researches on the anti-angiogenesis drugs in advanced breast cancer, the investigators believe that it is necessary to further explore the efficacy and safety of apatinib in advanced breast cancer.

**Detailed Description:-** With the comprehensive treatment of breast cancer wildly used in the clinical practice, the life quality of the patients with breast cancer has been improved greatly, and the survival of the patients has been extended as well.

However, the treatment of the patients with recurrent and metastatic breast cancer remains a major problem. There is still a lack of effective targeted therapy for Her-2 negative breast cancer.

Based on the present researches on the anti-angiogenesis drugs in advanced breast cancer, the investigators believe that it is necessary to further explore the efficacy and safety of apatinib in advanced breast cancer.

The aim of this research is to evaluate the progression-free survival (PFS) of the patients with HER-2 negative advanced breast cancer with chest wall metastasis in the treatment of apatinib.

**Location:-** China
Beijing Cancer Hospital
Beijing Beijing 100142 China

**Principal Investigator:-** Huiping Li, MD
**Tel:-** 010-4008-919191
**Email:-** huipingli2012@hotmail.com

**European Celecoxib Trial in Primary Breast Cancer (REACT).**

**Purpose:-** It has been found that the chemical changes that take place in a patient's body during the development of inflammation may provide an environment which stimulates cancer cells. One step in the development of inflammation is the production of certain chemical substances which are important in the formation and spread of tumors.

These are called prostaglandins. Cyclo-oxygenase II (COX-2) is an enzyme (a substance that speeds up chemical changes in the body) involved in the production of these prostaglandins and although it is not usually present in most tissues it is made at the sites of inflammation. Celecoxib is a selective Non-Steroidal Anti Inflammatory Drug (NSAID) which works by blocking the action of the COX-2 enzyme, leading to a decrease in the production of prostaglandins and a reduction in inflammation.

The purpose of this study is therefore to find out if celecoxib can be used after breast cancer treatment (chemotherapy and/ or radiotherapy) to reduce inflammation and thus reduce the ability of new tumors to grow and survive.

2590 women with primary breast cancer will be recruited in this study from several locations in the United Kingdom and Germany. Eligible patients will be randomly allocated a treatment group, which can be celecoxib or placebo.

Both treatments are taken orally (celecoxib 400mg daily, placebo 2 tablets daily) for a total of 2 years. In addition, hormone receptor positive patients will receive endocrine treatment as per local practice. Patients will prematurely discontinue treatment with celecoxib/placebo if disease progression is confirmed or if patients experience unacceptable toxicity.

Patients will be seen every 6 months for the first 3 years and then off treatment follow-up is carried out annually. Participating patients will also be given the option to take part in the pathology sub-study by donating a sample of the tumor tissue collected at the time of the primary surgery.

**Location:-** England
Imperial College London
Institute of Cancer Research, United Kingdom

**Principal Investigator:-** Charles R Coombes, MD
**Tel:-** +44 020 7594 9000
**Email:-** c.coombes@imperial.ac.uk

---

**Exemestane in Preventing Cancer in Postmenopausal Women at Increased Risk of Developing Breast Cancer.**

**Purpose:-** RATIONALE: The MAP.3 study was designed to test whether hormone therapy using exemestane may prevent breast cancer by blocking the production of estrogen. This study was analyzed in April 2011 and showed a 65% reduction in the incidence of invasive breast cancer in women receiving exemestane compared to women on placebo.

**PURPOSE:** The study protocol was amended in May 2011 and the current purpose of the study is to allow all study participants the opportunity to complete 5 years of exemestane.

**OBJECTIVES:-** Previously: To determine if exemestane reduces the incidence of invasive breast cancer compared with placebo.

**Location:-** Massachusetts - USA
Massachusetts General Hospital
55 Fruit Street Boston, MA 02114
**Principal Investigator:-** Paul E. Goss, MD, PhD
**Tel:-** 617-726-6500

**Email:-** pgoss@partners.org

---

**Chemotherapy-Induced Changes to Cognition and DNA in Breast Cancer Survivors.**

**Purpose:-** The purpose of this study is to learn more about how chemotherapy affects an individual's thinking abilities (cognition). Some research has shown that chemotherapy can cause changes in cognition in breast cancer survivors.

However, it is not clear why this change occurs. In this study, the investigators will look to see if damage to DNA is related to these changes in cognition. Specifically, the investigators want to see 1) if women who have been treated with chemotherapy have more DNA damage than healthy women; and 2) if DNA damage is related to cognitive problems in breast cancer survivors and healthy women.

**Detailed Description:-** The primary objective of this proposal is to obtain preliminary data regarding the association between DNA damage and cognitive functioning in breast cancer survivors. Specifically, we predict that:

**1.** Breast cancer survivors treated with chemotherapy and hormonal therapy will have higher levels of DNA damage as measured by the Comet assay as compared to age and education matched survivors treated with hormonal therapy only and healthy controls.

**2.** Survivors who meet criteria for cognitive impairment will have higher levels of DNA damage as compared to cancer survivors who do not meet criteria for cognitive impairment and healthy controls.
**Locations:-** United States, New York
Memorial Sloan Kettering Cancer Center at Commack
Commack, New York, United States

Memorial Sloan-Kettering Cancer Center, 1275 York Avenue, New York, NY 10021

Memorial Sloan Kettering Cancer Center at Mercy Medical Center
Rockville Centre, New York, United States, 11570

**Principal Investigator:-** Tim Ahles, PhD
**Tel:-** 212-639-2000 or 646-888-0200
**Email:-** ahlest@mskcc.org

---

## Phase IIB Neoadjuvant Enzalutamide (ZT) Plus Taxol for Androgen Receptor (AR)-Positive Triple-Negative Breast Cancer (AR+ TNBC).

**Purpose:-** The goal of this clinical research study is to learn if a combination of enzalutamide and paclitaxel can help to control triple-negative breast cancer (TNBC) by shrinking the tumors in the breast and/or lymph nodes before they are surgically removed. The safety of this treatment combination will also be studied.

**Primary Outcome Measures:-** Pathologic Complete Response (pCR) of Participants with Triple Negative Breast Cancer (TNBC) [Time Frame: 84 days].

At the end of 12 cycles, imaging scans of the breast and lymph nodes performed to check the status of the disease. Treatment worthy of further study if at least 4 of the 37 patients with pCR.

**Locations:-** United States, Texas
University of Texas MD Anderson Cancer Center
Houston, Texas, United States, 77030
**Principal Investigator:-** Naoto Ueno, MD, PhD
**Tel:-** 713-792-8754
**Email:-** nueno@mdanderson.org

# ALTERNATIVE BREAST CANCER Tx.

Cancer reversal is quite possible, but it requires some effort, some personal commitment and trust on the part of the others involved, and a comprehensive knowledge by the physician or alternative health practitioner of the modalities available and their effectiveness as proven in clinical practice.

Mortality from certain cancers may seem statistically likely, but that is an illusion compounded by fear and ignorance. It's not only patients who fear cancer outcomes; probably most oncologists are equally in fear of this disease and shield themselves against the disturbing scenarios, statistics, and probabilities they know too well.

The physician's treatments researched in this review offer patients the statistics of optimism. Men and women can and do survive cancer, and go on to live long, productive, healthy-lives—hopefully, cancer free.

We will now discuss most of the alternative treatments, examine dietary support, botanicals and supplements that fight cancer, and treatments for specifically neutralizing cancer and tumors.

There are many more additions to what we present and we hope that you will take action to win the battle over cancer by contacting a health professional to help you begin an alternative program, such as the physicians and centers listed at the end.

Here is an example of the cancer process and its reversal by the person most affected - a woman with breast cancer with metastases to the bones.

Lisa, aged 44, was a chemist with a lifelong habit of eating high-fat foods and pushing herself to workaholic extremes. She was a single mother of 3 children and worked full time. When she was diagnosed with breast cancer, she agreed to the orthodox strategy of surgery and chemotherapy.

After these treatments, she decided to forgo the radiation treatment the surgeon recommended because the chemotherapy had left her "feeling so weak." She thought having radiation would be too much for her system to handle. Three years late, the cancer returned with a vengeance, this time metastasizing to Lisa's bones.

A bone scan revealed that cancer had permeated both sides of her rib cage and seemed to be moving into her spine. Several specialists told her nothing could be done and that she probably had less than a year of life.

Now she had a difficult decision, whether to receive the same treatments as before and hope for the best, or should she look for ways to support the self-healing ability of her body through alternative treatments?

She visited Dr. Keith Block, M.D., mentioned along with other alternative physicians at the end of the review, the next month and found that his integrated system of nutrition, botanicals, phytochemicals, tailored exercise, and personalized stress management appealed to her. She was impressed with the variety of non-invasive and low-invasive methods intended to diminish side effects and boost effectiveness.

Within days of beginning Dr. Block's program, Lisa began to feel more energized and enthusiastic. Ten months into the program, her bone cancer was markedly reduced. For several months she continued to take an anti-estrogen drug (Tamoxifen), but later discontinued it with Dr. Block's approval due to harsh side effects.

Lisa followed his dietary and lifestyle advice, attending his intensive health education seminars in nutrition, cooking, therapeutic fitness, medicinal herbs, stress reduction, along with training sessions in nutrition, detoxification, meditation, imagery, cognitive restructuring, and personally tailored fitness techniques to strengthen her immune system.

Exercise and relaxation were vital aspects of her recovery. She practiced a series of slow, contemplative movements; which Dr. Block taught her, and she regularly walked and bicycled. She states that these were very relaxing to her and she did them frequently.

Lisa's efforts paid off in a huge way. After 16 months on the Block program, new CT and bone scans revealed that all of Lisa's cancer had disappeared. More than 13 years later, she feels better that ever and she says her life feels much more balanced.

---

## Therapies and Vaccines To Combat Breast Cancer:-

### T/Tn Antigen Breast Cancer Vaccine:-
Georg Springer, M.D., showed that 2 antigens, called T and Tn, play a vital role in the immune system's ability to respond to cancer and are present in 90% of all cancers. Through the use of a specially developed vaccine, Dr. Springer demonstrated that the immune system's reaction to T and Tn antigens results in strong cancer cell killing activity.

Cancer cells have proteins, or antigens, on their surfaces that can be recognized by the immune system. The identification of certain cancer-related antigens forms the basis for the exciting approach embraced by Georg Springer, M.D. Dr. Springer is an immunologist who founded the Heather Bligh Cancer Research Laboratories at the Chicago Medical School. This pioneering German scientist-physician has shown that 2 antigens, called T and Tn, play a vital role in the immune system's ability to respond to cancer. Since the early 1980's, Dr. Springer has repeatedly shown that the immune system's reaction to T and Tn antigens results in strong cancer cell killing activity in both animal and human studies.

Using various biochemical tests, Dr. Springer has detected the T and Tn antigens in over 90% of all cancers. The less aggressive cancer (meaning they are well differentiated) produce a higher proportion of the T antigen, while the Tn antigen predominates in the more aggressive cancers (meaning they are poorly differentiated). The overall concentrations of the T and Tn antigens correlate with the aggressiveness of breast cancer,

In 1974, Dr. Springer had his first opportunity to test his experimental vaccine when his wife, Heather Bligh, developed breast cancer, and was told she had only a year to live. After receiving the T/Tn vaccine, however, she lived a full 6 years.

Encouraged, Dr. Springer began, a pilot study with 19 breast cancer patients, all of whom went on to survive at least 5 years on the T/TN vaccine; 16 of these women (84%) are still alive, I I of them after a decade or more of their supposedly terminal diagnosis.

In another study, 26 women with advanced breast cancer (10 with Stage IV, 6 Stage III, 10 Stage II cancers) were given the T/Tn vaccine after undergoing an operation for their primary cancer or after the first recurrence.

All survived over 5 years, and only 5 out of the 26 patients died within 5-10 years from the time of vaccination; 14 of 18 patients (78%) who were vaccinated over 10 years ago are still alive, and half of these long-term survivors have lived longer than 18 years since their operation." An additional 49 breast cancer patients have been vaccinated since 1994 and are being closely monitored by Dr. Springer and his colleagues.

Once breast cancer has spread to the bone or to a distant organ (Stage III or Stage IV cancer), only 10% of cancer patients on conventional treatment survive 5 years. In contrast, breast cancer patients who receive Dr. Springer's T/Tn vaccine have shown a clearly superior survival advantage. "A great number of our patients have been well-publicized."

Dr. Springer emphasizes that nutritional support is also important. He advises his patients to take, once daily, a multivitamin, vitamin C (3-4 g), beta carotene (20,000 IU) and vitamin E (1600 IU).

Maurice Black at New York Medical College's Institute of Breast Diseases found that Stage II patients with compromised immune systems cut their five-year risk of a recurrence from 38 % to 6 % by taking vitamin E. "The nutritional component is extremely important because nutrients have been shown to influence both cell-mediated and antibody facets of the immune response," says Dr. Springer. "I recommend that my patients consume a wholesome, high-fiber diet that includes fish and liver to obtain the beneficial nutrients from these foods."

In theory, says Dr. Springer, his immune-stimulating vaccine could be used for the treatment of all cancers. "Breast cancer serves as our model for treating all carcinomas, which make up about 85% of all lethal cancers. Most importantly, we may be able to prevent all these cancers using the vaccine." However, since the T antigen has not been found in brain tumors or in sarcomas (bone and muscle), the vaccine is unlikely to have any therapeutic impact on these cancers.

---

**Immuno-Augmentative Therapy:-**
A biologist and cancer researcher named Lawrence Burton, Ph.D., has developed an alternative cancer therapy called IAT. He identified and isolated blood protein components that he suspected were associated

with the development of cancer. One of these, called C3 complement, activates two tumor antibodies, one is a deblocking protein factor.

According to his theory, when the four blood components are balanced, the body can subdue cancer cells as part of its normal activity, if any of them are not balanced, the body's cancer defenses drop.

He discovered that by injecting certain amounts of these components into the patients, remissions of many types of cancer would occur, including some labeled as terminal.

It is not a cure for cancer, however, it is more like a controller of cancer, and much like insulin is for diabetes. IAT has achieved tumor reduction and even complete remission according to Dr Burton in 40 to 60% of the patients who received it.

Since IAT is builds on the body's anticancer immune function, it is virtually nontoxic. The survival rate of Dr. Burton's patients was approximately double the maximum survival rate of conventionally treated patients who had metatstatic cancers, from a study he completed of 79 patients with advanced cancers. For more information on Immuno Augmentative Therapy, contact the IAT Center, PO Box F-42689, Freeport, Grand Bahama, Telephone: 242-352-4755.

In the normal healthy person any mutant cancer cells are recognized and antibodies attempt to destroy them; this reaction is promoted by **Tumor Complement** (TC), which is produced by cancer cells, and is the effective signal to the antibodies to destroy that cell. These necrotic tumor cells are then passed to the liver to be "sanitized." If Tumor cell necrosis occurs too rapidly the liver can be overloaded, leading to production of blocking Proteins which shield Tumor cells and slows down the antibody reaction to those cells. Patients with cancer may have very high levels of this Blocking Protein. Deblocking Proteins neutralize this blocking action and so enable antibodies to access the Tumor cells. Patients with cancer tend to have a deficiency of Deblocking Protein.

In order to effect this control you need Tumor Complement produced by the cancer cell to alert and activate the Antibodies and you also need sufficient Deblocking Protein to neutralize the Blocking Protein and allow the antibodies access to the cancer cells.

Deblocking Protein (DP) —an alpha 2 macroglobulin derive from the pooled sera of healthy donors. (In usual scientific use, alpha 2 macroglobulin would refer to an antibody belonging to one of the five major classes of bloodborne immunoglobulin, the Ig M group. Although Burton describes DP as an alpha 2 macroglobulin, to OTA's knowledge he has produced no analytical results to confirm that. No alpha 2 macroglobulin that has been identified by mainstream researchers has the properties Burton ascribes to DP.)

Burton states that treatment regimens are based on his determination of the patient's initial immunocompetence and the responses of past patients with similar status, which have been compiled in a computer program.

As therapy proceeds, Burton tests patients' blood daily or twice-daily for the relative concentrations of four basic factors: Tumor Antibody (TA1 and TA2), Tumor Complement (TC), Blocking Protein Factor (BPF), and Deblocking Protein Factor (DPF). BPF "blocks" the claimed anti-tumor effects of TA1 and TA2, and is not administered as part of the IAT regimen.

Burton adjusts the daily prescription of TA1, TA2, TC and DPF in light of his blood tests during patients' initial six- to eight-week course. Patients inject themselves subcutaneously or intramuscularly with the prescribed amounts. Other medications (e.g., prednisone, a corticosteroid) are also prescribed for many patients.

Tumor antibodies are "**alerted to the presence**" of tumor cells by a protein produced by the tumor cells themselves-**tumor complement factor.** Tumor complement induces the tumor antibodies to destroy the tumor cells. If the tumor cells are destroyed in an unregulated manner, however, a person's liver may become overburdened.

To protect the body, blocking protein factors are produced to shield the tumor cells from attack by the tumor antibodies and thereby regulate the rate of tumor kill. The important balance of tumor kill rate is maintained by yet another blood component-de-blocking protein factor which neutralizes the blocking protein and thereby permits antibodies to destroy tumor cells in a regulated manner.

At times this dynamic process is upset and an over-supply of blocking protein factor exists, along with undersupplies of deblocking protein factors and tumor complement factor. When this imbalance occurs, the individual is said to be **immuno-suppressed** or **immunodeficient.**

According to his brochure, Burton's laboratory made daily or twice-daily assessments of the levels and proportions of "**tumor complement**," "tumor antibody," "**deblocking protein**," and "**blocking proteins**."

The patient was then given daily injections of "tumor complement factor" obtained from the serum of persons with cancer and "deblocking protein factor" and "tumor antibody" obtained from the serum of persons without cancer. Burton determined the dosages after analyzing these data with a computer program that he developed.

Saul Green, Ph.D., a biochemist who did cancer research at Memorial Sloan-Kettering Hospital for 23 years, has examined the patent applications. Dr. Green concluded that Burton's postulated "tumor complement," "tumor antibody," "deblocking protein," and "blocking proteins" in fact, have "never been identified as components of human blood much less of the immune system in the human."

Moreover, proteins with the molecular weights Burton attributes to these alleged substances cannot be separated by centrifugation of blood using the speeds and times described in his patents. A report to the OTA reached similar conclusions.

Dr. Green also noted that Burton did not establish immunologic baselines for normal individuals that were verified by independent investigators. Nor did he use recognized scientific tests to determine the status of his patients' immune competence either before or after treatment.

## TVZ-7 Lymphocyte Treatment:-

TVZ-7 is an example of a specific immunotherapy. This technique consists of culturing and harvesting B-lymphocytes, a form of white blood cells that produce antibodies, which neutralize foreign and dangerous matter in the blood.

The extracted material, consisting of immune molecules, which include interferons, interleukins and tumor necrosis factor, are called TVZ-7, and is administered intravenously in 44-50 treatments during two weeks. Canadian physicians, who see remarkable results with cancers of the blood, pancreas, skin, reproductive organs, colon, liver brain and gallbladder, utilize it mainly in other countries and. Hormonally responsive tumors, such as those of the breast, seem to respond especially well.

For more information on TVZ-7, contact Integrated Biologics Ltd.,

Biotechnology Research and Development. 130 Commerce Way, Woburn, MA 01801, Telephone 617-938-9088 and Dr. Ravi Devgan of Ontario, Canada at 416-487-0882.

---

**Autogenous Bacterial Vaccine:-**
This is based on a form-changing microbe identified by Virginia Livingston, M.D. called *P.cryptocides*, which is found in high concentrations in cancer patients.

It is described by her as a hidden killer and a lethal bloodstream infection that shows no direct signs of its existence. She developed a way to administer a vaccine made from the patient's own bacteria to fight this cancer microbe.

It is normally present in everyone, but is kept at bay by the immune system. When poor diet, stress, chemical toxins, and many other factors suppress immunity, what normally is a dormant microbe can multiply and promote the growth of tumors. This microbe was identified in very high concentrations in cancer patients.

This vaccine is made by the bacteria in the person's body and fights the same bacteria; therefore the vaccine precisely matches each individual. They also contain vitamins and minerals to strengthen the immune system. It is given every 3 to 5 days, depending on the patient.

Other researchers report positive results with the Livingston vaccines, with no adverse reaction except for an occasional rash.

For more information on this, contact The Livingston Foundation Medical Center 3232 Duke Street, San Diego, CA 92110, and Telephone 619-224-3515.

**Immuno-Placental Therapy (IPT):-**

This therapy was pioneered by Russian immunologist Valentine I. Govallo, M.D. He is the director of the Moscow Medical Institute's Laboratory of Clinical Immunology.

The premise is that cancer had a specific immunologic character that allows it to evade attack by the human immune system. Dr. Govallo discovered that this special factor is found in the human placenta, and he developed a vaccine from placental blood after live human birth to give the cancer patient's immune system the ability to overpower the cancer and its "**cloaking device**."

Other vaccines are very specific to certain types of cancer. Sometimes the body's same ability to cause tumor cells to die may also turn off the body's immune response to foreign tissues. In these cases tumor cells can gain advantage over the anti-cancer responses of the body.

Dr. Govallo's vaccine takes the human placenta factors that appear to suppress the defense mechanism of malignant cells, effectively allowing the tumor to be attacked and killed off.

His approach is called IPT, but is widely known asVG-1000. It has been used effectively in the treatment of advanced cancers, with survival rates noted from his studies of over 20 years. IPT seems particularly effective for breast cancer.

The only side effect seems to be an occasional fever and fatigue for 1-2 days. It is not indicated for the treatment of liver cancer, but is highly effective for most forms of early and advanced cancers. Dr Govallo's placental vaccine is available at Max Gerson Memorial Center Hospital in

Tijuana, Mexico, and IAT in Freeport, Bahamas. Contact People Against Cancer, Box 10, Otho, IA 50569, Telephone 515-972-4444 for more information.

---

**Injectable Substances Which Combat Breast Cancer:-**

**Ukrain**

This substance is derived from a combination of a common weed called clendine (chelidonium majus) and thiophosphoric acid, one of the original chemotherapeutic agents. This combination appears to neutralize the toxic effect of the alkaloids contained the plant.

By this method, Ukrain has been rendered almost completely nontoxic, and fortified the body's tissues and anticancer defenses. It is a potent anticancer agent and also very safe. Like chemotherapy, it kills cancer cells very well, but unlike chemotherapy, it spares normal, healthy tissue.

"Ukrain appears to halt cancer growth by interfering with oxygen respiration in cancer cells. Success rates with Ukrain in cancer are best in the early stages: 93% and 72% in Stages I and II, and 30% for advanced metastatic cancer.

Laboratory testing to date indicates Ukrain can affect even cancers such as brain, lung and melanoma. This information comes from a 10 year study at the Ukrainian Anti-Cancer Institute in Vienna."

Ukrain can be purchased from Nowicky Pharma Margaretenstrasse 7 A-1040 Vienna, Austria. Telephone # 011 43 1 586 1224 Fax 011 43 1 586 8994. Speak with Mr. Hodish, who speaks understandable English. Email:- nowicky@ukrin.com or go to their site http://www.ukrin.com

Ukrain should not be used with the drug Dexamethason (Dacradron) because it contains cortisone, which neutralizes the Ukrain.

---

**Amygdalin/Laetrile:-**
This substance is highly concentrated in the pits of apricots, peaches, cherries, and berries. It is one of a group called nitrilosides, and has been found to have strong cancer-fighting potential, particularly with regard to secondary cancers, including a 60% reduction in lung metastases.

It appears to neutralize the oxidative cancer-promoting compounds such as free radicals, which is just one more key component for keeping cancer from growing or spreading, and is considered entirely safe to use, also its one of the best known, and most proven, cancer treatment on earth. It has been severely suppressed by our government, which has even reached into Mexico to stop this treatment!

Although Laetrile may possibly be safe, at least if used in small doses, scientific results do not support its effectiveness.

Laetrile (the chemical amygdalin) is found in the kernels of many fruits, notably apricots, peaches, plums and bitter almonds. It is also found in cassava, lima beans and numerous other plants in a slightly different chemical form.

The notion of using Laetrile as a cancer drug got its first major impetus in the United States in 1920 when Ernst T. Krebs Sr., a California physician, tried apricot pits as a cancer treatment. Laetrile received another big shove in 1952 when Ernst T. Krebs Jr., a biochemist, developed a purified form of Laetrile for injection.

Yet only in recent years, and especially during the past few months, have thousands of Americans been clamoring for Laetrile, largely through the promotion of organizations such as the Committee for Freedom of Choice in Cancer Therapy and the National Health Foundation.

Some Laetrile proponents have been pushing the U.S. Food and Drug Administration to approve it. The FDA has resisted on the grounds that Laetrile is worthless against cancer.

Other Laetrile supporters have tried to get around FDA prohibition of interstate commerce of Laetrile by smuggling it into the United States from Mexico or by legalizing its manufacture and use on a state-by-state basis. So far they have made headway, particularly in the latter direction. Seven states have approved Laetrile use.

The Laetrile controversy seems to keep growing. Should Americans be allowed to use the drug or not? Not enough attention, however, has been devoted to the science behind Laetrile. What evidence is there for the safety of Laetrile and for its effectiveness against cancer? Is the evidence sufficient to pass judgment on Laetrile as a cancer drug?

The first and somewhat easier question is that of Laetrile's safety. Extensive animal experiments on the safety and effectiveness of Laetrile were conducted by a team of researchers at the Memorial Sloan-Kettering Cancer Center in New York City and at the Catholic Medical Center in Woodhaven, N.Y., from 1972 to 1976, and the results will be published early next year in the Journal of Surgical Oncology.

These experiments showed no harmful effects of Laetrile in mice except when very large doses were used. Nor when Laetrile was given along with accepted cancer drugs did it alter their benefits or toxicity.

Exactly how much Laetrile is safe for humans, however, has really not been determined, and certainly it can be harmful if taken in sufficient doses. For instance, two cancer patients were treated for serious adverse reactions to Laetrile last month at the Georgetown University Medical Center in Washington. One of the patients developed fever, rash and gastrointestinal symptoms that promptly disappeared after discontinuation of Laetrile, only to recur after she resumed taking the compound.

The other patient experienced a weakening of the eye muscles and eyelids. Within 48 hours of being taken off Laetrile, his condition improved dramatically and resolved itself completely within six days.

Then in June, a Buffalo, N.Y., infant died from accidental ingestion of an unknown number of Laetrile pills her father was taking. (Laetrile ultimately breaks down in the body into the poison cyanide.) Several Californians who ate apricot pits as a health food suffered cyanide poisoning from them. A three-year-old girl who ate 15 apricot kernels experienced cyanide poisoning as well. Both acute and chronic cyanide poisoning have been reported among Nigerians, Jamaicans and Malasians who ate a lot of cassava.

As for Laetrile's effectiveness, or lack thereof, the evidence is more extensive and complex. First the test-tube evidence:

Unlike many cancer remedies of questionable value, Laetrile is a well-known and identifiable chemical substance, amygdalin. Amygdalin is broken down in the body by enzymes known as beta-glucosidases to yield dextrose and mandelonitrile, which is benzyaldehyde plus a molecule of hydrogen cyanide. Laetrile proponents offer several different arguments for how Laetrile's pharmacological actions can kill cancer tissues in the body.

One of their arguments, initiated by Ernst Krebs Jr., is that cancer tissues are selectively killed by Laetrile because they contain more of the beta-glucosidase enzymes than healthy tissues do. Is there any scientific basis to this claim?

Evidently not. As Joseph R. DiPalma, professor of pharmacology at Hahnemann Medical College in Philadelphia, told SCIENCE NEWS, "Cancer cells which have been analyzed many, many times have very little contents of this type of enzymes." Thomas H. Jukes, a nutrition scientist at the University of California at Berkeley, agreed in the Sept. 13, 1976, JOURNAL OF THE AMERICAN MEDICAL ASSOCIATION: "There are only traces of beta-glucosidase in animal tissues and even less in experimental tumors?"

Another Laetrilist claim is that rhodanese, an enzyme that converts toxic hydrogen cyanide to nontoxic thiocyanate, is present in tumors in lower amounts than it is present in normal tissues, and hence tumors cannot protect themselves against hydrogen cyanide. Is there any basis to this argument? It doesn't look like it.

According to Daniel S. Martin, a cancer-therapy scientist at the Catholic Medical Center and one of the investigators in the recent Laetrile studies at that complex, assays of this enzyme have shown no such differences between cancerous and healthy tissues.

Still a third assertion by Laetrile proponents is that Laetrile is a vitamin--vitamin B and thus a nutritional substance rather than a drug. Is there any evidence to support this claim? Dean Burk, a former National Cancer Institute scientist, believes that there might be.

He asserts that it is "almost impossible ever to declare scientifically that a given compound is not a vitamin" and that "meats, milk, cheese, eggs and other proteins may similarly produce cyanide when decomposed by suitable enzymes or catalysts."

In contrast, Jukes declares that Laetrile has "not the slightest resemblance to a vitamin. The crucial property of a vitamin is that its absence from the diet produces a specific deficiency disease in vertebrate animals. The cyanogenetic glycosides do not have this property."

Yet when SCIENCE NEWS asked DiPalma whether tests had ever been conducted to determine whether Laetrile's absence from the diet might cause a deficiency disease, he replied: "I believe it is very easy to fall into the trap of trying to disprove something which has not enough merit to be disproven in the first place.

Obviously the great majority of the world's population does not consume amygdalin in any form, and it is ridiculous to even suggest that Laetrile is a vitamin."

So Laetrile has really not been adequately tested to determine whether it is a vitamin or not. Even if Laetrile were found to be a vitamin, of course, its vitamin properties would not demonstrate that it is also effective against tumors. Only one other vitamin has shown any anticancer properties to date, and that is vitamin A (SN: 3/13/76, p. 165).

Taking all of the above test-tube evidence into consideration, then, the conclusion is that none of it supports the ability of Laetrile to kill tumors.

Do animal experiments with Laetrile indicate any effectiveness against cancer? Take those conducted at the National Cancer Institute or under NCI contract at other institutions.

The first was conducted at the Warf Institute in Madison, Wis., under NCI contract, in 1957. Laetrile was given to mice that had had tumors transplanted onto them--a common system for screening compounds for anticancer activity. Although the results of this experiment were not published, they showed that Laetrile produced no significant inhibition of tumor growth nor a significant increase in lifespan in the mice that had been given cancer. In 1960, a second experiment was run, under NCI contract, at Microbiological Associates, Inc.

This time Laetrile from a different source was tested against the same mouse tumors. Again no anti-tumor activity was found. The results were not published.

Then in 1969, a third Laetrile test was conducted at Microbiological Associates. This time Laetrile was tested alone or in combination with the enzyme that helps break it down in the body, beta-glucosidase, against leukemia in mice.

The results, which were not published, showed that Laetrile was ineffective against cancer, either alone or in combination with the enzyme.

A fourth Laetrile experiment was carried out in 1973, under NCI contract, by Isidore Wodinsky and Joseph K. Swinarski of Arthur D. Little, Inc. of Cambridge, Mass. Laetrile, in daily injections of 3,200 milligrams per kilogram of body weight down to 6.25 mg/kg, was tested alone or in combination with beta-glucosidase against four kinds of tumors in rodents. It was found ineffective alone or in combination with the enzyme.

These results were published in the September/October 1975 CANCER CHEMOTHERAPY REPORTS. A fifth experiment was conducted, under NCI contract, by W.R. Laster Jr. and F.M. Schabel Jr. of the Southern Research Institute in Birmingham, Ala. Laetrile, in injections of 500 mg/kg of body weight down to 23 mg/kg was tested alone or in combination with beta-glucosidase against three transplanted mouse tumors.

No anti-tumor activity was found. These results were also published in the September/ October 1975 Cancer Chemotherapy Reports.

Finally a sixth experiment has just been completed, under NCI contract, at the Battelle Memorial Institute in Columbus, Ohio, by David P. Houchens and Artemio A. Ovejera. In one phase, mice with breast cancer or colon cancer were injected every four days with three doses of 400, 800 or 1,600 mg/kg body weight of Laetrile.

In another phase, mice with colon cancer were divided into separate groups and treated for nine days with either Laetrile alone; beta-glucosidase, the enzyme that breaks Laetrile down in the body into cyanide; or Laetrile and beta-glucosidase.

The scientists report that they found no difference in the growth of the tumors that they followed for 42 days in the mice that did and did not receive Laetrile.

Thus NCI or NCI-sponsored Laetrile animal experiments concur with the test-tube evidence to date that Laetrile has no anticancer activity.

The most extensive animal tests ever conducted on the substance in the United States were done at Sloan-Kettering and the Catholic Medical Center. The Sloan-Kettering investigators included C. Chester Stock, George S. Tarnowski, Franz A. Schmid, Dorris J. Hutchison, Morris H. Teller, Kanematsu Sugiura, Isabel M. Mountain and Elisabeth Stockert. The Catholic Medical Center investigators were Daniel S. Martin and Ruth A. Fugman.

Eleven series of experiments, 23 experiments all told, were conducted to determine whether Laetrile has any ability to counter spontaneous breast cancer or leukemia in mice.

The cd sub8 f sub 1 strain of mice was used in most of the breast-cancer research, the Swiss Webster albino mouse strain from one breast-cancer study and the AKR mice for the leukemia studies. Nineteen of the studies were performed with Laetrile obtained from Mexico, the other four with Laetrile from Germany.

The doses of Laetrile used in all but two of the experiments varied from 1,000 to 3,000 mg/kg of body weight, considerably more than Laetrile patients usually take. In one experiment, 40 mg/kg of Laetrile was employed, which more closely approximated the 3 grams a day taken by many Laetrile patients.

In the other experiment, doses as high as 4,000 and 5,000 mg/kg were used. Results from all the studies suggested that neither the source of Laetrile nor the dose level used produce any great differences in outcome. However, there were some discrepancies among the study results, apparently due to another cause.

In the initial set of six experiments, for instance, Suguira gave Laetrile to 60 mice and saline injections to 60 control mice. He found that while 90 percent of the control mice experienced lung metastases due to spreading breast tumors, only 21 percent of the treated mice did.

Thus the investigators at Sloan-Kettering and the Catholic Medical Center conducted the subsequent experiments to see whether they could confirm these initial promising results and perhaps even expand them.

Partial confirmation was achieved in a joint experiment conducted by Suguira and Schmid. Whereas Suguira noted lung metastases among 100 percent of control mice, he noted only 38 percent among treated mice. Whereas Schmid identified 80 percent of control mice with metastases, he identified only 44 percent of treated mice with them.

In fact, Suguira confirmed his initial results with two other experiments he conducted alone. In one, 91 percent of control mice showed metastases, versus 22 percent of the treated mice. In the other, 81 percent of controls showed metastases, versus only 17 percent of treated mice.

However, in the numerous other experiments conducted with or without Suguira, the investigators were not able to approach these promising results and in several instances even came up with better results for controls than for treated animals.

For example, in an experiment on mice with spontaneous breast cancer that he conducted alone, Schmid found lung metastases among 70 percent of treated mice versus only 58 percent for controls.

In a joint experiment on mice with spontaneous breast tumors, Martin, Fugman, Tarnowski and Suguira found lung metastases in 42 percent of the treated mice versus 21 percent of the controls.

Why such a discrepancy in results? Apparently it is because not all of the experiments were evaluated by the same method. Results favorable to Laetrile nearly all resulted from macrovision or microscopic examination and mostly from Suguira's visual observation at that.

 The results most unfavorable to Laetrile came from bioassay, where lungs from the test animals were shredded and injected into other mice. If the lung tissue injections made tumors form, then one could conclude that the lungs had contained metastases.

A prime example of how these two methods of evaluation produced discrepant results came from a blind experiment on spontaneous breast cancers in mice conducted by Suguira. In this arrangement, he did not know which of the mice had received Laetrile and which had not.

Suguira's visual evaluation showed that 54 percent of the treated mice experienced lung metastases compared with 63 percent of control mice. Bioassay, in contrast, demonstrated that 85 percent of the treated mice, compared with 83 percent of control mice, were positive for them. In still another blind experiment conducted by Suguira, visual evaluation produced somewhat favorable results for Laetrile; bioassay did not.

Which type of evaluation is one to believe, then? The bioassay results must be considered the stronger of the two since they are totally objective. There is no need to rely on an observer's eyesight or unintentional visual bias, which is the case with macrovision or microscopic examination.

In other words, Suguira's positive results for Laetrile, dependent entirely on visual observation, could be pitted against the less favorable visual results obtained by the other investigators, but they simply cannot stack up against the negative results procured by bioassay.

When all these results are taken together, then, they, like the NCI animal tests and test-tube research, rule out anticancer activity for Laetrile. What's more, the Sloan-Kettering investigators tested Laetrile against various kinds of transplanted tumors in mice. These results were totally negative.

Finally, how about clinical evidence for Laetrile's effectiveness against tumors? Some 50,000 Americans have so far taken Laetrile for cancer. A number of them have not been helped by it or even have died. Yet other attest to Laetrile's curative powers or at least to its palliative effects—i.e. pain relief or feeling better.

Do such testimonials constitute clinical evidence for Laetrile's efficacy? No, most cancer scientists reply. For instance, in many cases where patients have claimed that Laetrile has brought about a cancer remission, pathology reports have not been available to document the before and after effects or even that a patient had cancer in the first place.

As for Laetrile's palliative effects, scientists tend to point out that they are probably psychologically induced and that such a placebo effect could be achieved with any drug in which a patient believes. Yet, even if Laetrile's pain-relieving impact were physiologically rather than psychologically induced, it would not be the same as antitumor activity.

So should a scientifically controlled clinical trial be conducted to test Laetrile's effectiveness against cancer? From a scientific viewpoint, no. All of the 40 anticancer drugs on the American market were shown to be active against tumors in animals before they were shown effective against human cancers.

In contrast, animal studies to date do not demonstrate antitumor activity for Laetrile. So it is highly unlikely that Laetrile would show any anticancer efficacy in a clinical trial. However, because of strong political pressure on the scientific community to conduct such a trial, the NCI may break precedence and do so.

Whether even a well-conducted clinical study would quell the Laetrile controversy, of course, is questionable in view of the antiscience, antiestablishment bias of many Laetrile proponents (see accompanying box). But then medical science would at least have done all that it could in order to arrive at a fair conclusion.

---

**The Laetrile controversy: Not just a science issue.**

The dispute over whether Laetrile should be legalized or not extends far beyond scientific evidence regarding its safety and efficacy. The best way to understand the issues is to examine the positions of Laetrile proponents and opponents.

One group of Laetrile supporters, members of the Committee for Freedom of Choice in Cancer Therapy, believes that cancer patients should have access to any drug they choose regardless of what the FDA rules.

A similar position is taken by members of the National Health Federation who advocate, along with Laetrile, other "natural" methods of healing such as health foods, chiropractic and acupuncture therapy.

In his book Health Purifiers and Their Enemies (Prodist 1977), Julius A. Roth writes: "Health freedom is essential to all these organizations. Its ideological essence is the ready possibility, open to us all, to choose whatever form of health maintenance or health care we wish."

Other Laetrile backers are political extremists of both left and right who deeply distrust the "establishment," whether it is political, medical or whatever.

They suspect that cancer researchers have covered up results that support Laetrile because the scientists have sold out to drug companies which cannot make money off of natural substances such as Laetrile and which hence do not want to see it marketed.

They are convinced that physicians oppose Laetrile because it would cure cancer patients and hence deprive them of doctor fees. For instance, at an FDA Laetrile hearing in May, John Yarbro, a physician at the University of Missouri School of Medicine, asked, "Do you really believe that a quarter-million physicians across this country could let people die so that they can make a profit?" Laetrile advocates clapped and jeered, "You said it! You said it! You said it!"

Yet some Laetrile champions appear to be out for a quick buck themselves. Some 7,000 cancer patients will undergo Laetrile treatments at two Tijuana, Mexico, clinics this year at an average weekly cost of $350. Customs officials on the Mexican border are seizing 40,000 vials of Laetrile monthly, making it the second biggest American smuggling problem after narcotics.

Laetrile now has a higher markup than heroin. Whether Laetrile legalization would benefit such profiteers is doubtful. However it would unquestionably fill the coffers of American Laetrile manufacturers and dispensers.

As for the Laetrile antagonists, such as the FDA, the American Cancer Society and most cancer scientists, they largely oppose the legalization of Laetrile on the grounds that it has not been shown effective against cancer and that the FDA requires that a drug must be shown not only safe but effective before it can be marketed. They claim that if an exception is made for Laetrile, it would erode the FDA's jurisdiction over other drugs.

They also argue that if Laetrile were made available to cancer patients, the patients would probably forego lifesaving cancer treatments and take Laetrile instead.

Given the radically different stances and motives of various Laetrile supporters and detractors, then, and particularly the antiscience, antiestablishment bias of many backers, it is highly unlikely that the present scientific evidence on Laetrile or even a clinical study of the drug will resolve the question of whether Laetrile should be legalized or not.

Rather, the issue will probably be decided by which group garners the most influence with Congress.

## Tissue Extracts:-

When taken orally or by injection, glandular and organ tissue extracts migrate directly to the gland or organ from which they are derived to provide support to that particular area and to help it fulfill its body-regulating and balancing functions.

Thymus extracts in particular, containing the thymus hormone called thymosin, have demonstrated effectiveness in treating cancers in both human and animal studies. In an animal study of lung cancer, a combination of thymosin and interferon (a natural immune system secretion) caused a "dramatic and rapid disappearance of tumor burden.

The animals treated with thymosin had stronger natural killer cell activity and lived significantly longer than those receiving standard chemotherapy.

In trials involving people with lung cancer, patients receiving thymosin had significantly prolonged survival times relative to the other treatment groups.

## Fibrocystic Breast Disease...Or Is It?

The term "**fibrocystic breast disease**" (FBD) is still widely used even though it does not represent either a distinct clinical or pathological entity. This term, along with synonyms such as "chronic cystic mastiffs" and "mammary dysplasia" is used to describe a benign condition characterized by cyclically fluctuating palpable irregularity of the breast tissue accompanied by swelling, pain, tenderness that fluctuates with the menstrual cycle.

The controversy exists as to whether or not the condition constitutes a disease process because the defining characteristics are present in 50% of all women clinically and 90% histologically.

Many think that these palpable lumps probably represent physiologic changes rather than a pathologic process. Pathologically, the changes included under the heading of fibrocystic disease include macroscopic and microscopic cysts, stromal fibrosis, apocrine metaplasia, and a variety of proliferative lesions. Since these changes are ubiquitous in female breasts, it may be misleading to diagnose this condition as a disease.

The significance of "fibrocystic disease" has been attributed to its possible relation to an increased incidence of developing breast cancer. However, several studies have clearly demonstrated that the relative risk is only related to which of the histologic subgroups are present.

The classification system for benign breast lesions of Dupont and Page separates the various components of fibrocystic disease into three groups, with different relative risks for the subsequent development of breast cancer: nonproliferative lesions, proliferative lesions without atypia, and atypical hyperplasias.

In their study, the only patients in the nonproliferative category with an increased risk of developing breast cancer were those with gross cysts plus a family history of breast cancer.

In the patients with proliferative lesions without atypia the risk was only slightly higher when they had a positive family history. Atypical hyperplasias are proliferative lesions that possess some of the features of carcinoma in situ. Atypical hyperplasias are categorized as either ductal or lobular.

In the study of Dupont and Page, patients with atypical hyperplasia had a significantly increased risk of developing breast cancer. Among the patients with atypical hyperplasia who also had a family history of breast cancer, the risk was even greater, approaching that of patients with carcinoma in situ.

The cause of FBD remains unknown although most researchers agree that ovarian hormones are implicated. They do not agree, however, as to whether or not FBD is an indication of abnormal hormone production or an exaggerated response to normal hormone levels by hypersensitive tissues.

Many investigators and clinicians and patients, also attribute a causative role to **methylxanthines** (a closely related group of alkaloids that includes caffeine).

The methylxanthines act as competitive inhibitors of the enzyme that breaks down cyclic adenosine monophosphate (cAMP), therefore an increase in methylxanthines causes an increase in cAMP. Women with FBD have been found to have statistically significant higher levels of cAMP in their breast tissue.

FBD is most common in women of about 40 years of age and more common in nulliparous women. FBD occurs more frequently in women with early menarche, late menopause, and irregular or anovulatory cycles. Women with FBD also are more likely to suffer from PMS. FBD tends to be a progressive condition if not attended to. Symptoms tend to increase and continue for longer time periods as women age, up until the menopause.

When giving a breast exam, check each breast for a rise or irregularity without a symmetric counterpart. Palpation reveals an area that is firmer than surrounding tissue, slightly irregular, tender, and generally mobile. A similar area palpated in the same quadrant in the other breast is generally a comforting finding.

Any single, unilateral dominant nodule is considered a critical finding and must be appropriately worked up. Any dominant solid mass that persists through a menstrual cycle mandates further evaluation regardless of mammographic findings.

Conventional management is most often achieved by hormone manipulation via pharmacological intervention. Oral contraceptives have been found to relieve FBD symptoms in 90% of women within three to six months of treatment, with 80% experiencing less tenderness after only one month of therapy.

**Progestins** have been used to correct the estrogen/progestin ratio of luteal insufficiency that is thought to be implicated in FBD. Administering 10 mg of medroxyprogesterone acetate on days 15 through 25 relieves symptoms in 80-85% of the patients with FBD. Continued use for three to four months generally brings marked improvement, although symptoms are not relieved permanently and weight gain and depression are fairly common.

**Danazol** and **Bromocriptine** therapy have also yielded 80-90% improvement but the side effects of these drugs make them generally unacceptable solutions.

The natural medicine approach to fibrocystic breast disease might first be to rename it **"fibrocystic changes"** as well as to offer both preventive measures and drugless therapeutics.

Most practitioners of alternative medicine as well as patients, have observed a relationship between caffeine and FBD. Researchers in some studies have found symptomatic improvement in subjects who reduced cafffeine, while other studies have found no changes and one study showed that symptoms worsened.

The use of vitamin E has probably been the most studied supplement for FBD. Vitamin E appears to regulate the synthesis of specific proteins and enzymes required in tissue differentiation. Doses of 600 IU daily were found subjectively and objectively beneficial in some studies.

Improving dietary habits to decrease estrogen sources in the diet, increasing fiber and following a low fat diet regime would be the hallmarks of a therapeutic diet for FBD.

Additional therapeutic plans often include **evening primrose oil, beta carotene, iodine, methionine, B-complex, choline, and/or flaxseed oil**, depending on the individual case and the response to simple dietary changes, the avoidance of caffeine and supplementing vitamin E.

Botanical diuretics are successfully used to decrease premenstrual fluid engorgement of the breasts.

It seems the best choice is the **Taraxacum leaf**. Botanical formulations are also successfully used to restore proper hormonal balance. Botanicals such as **Foeniculum, Angelica, Macrotys, and Arctium** are observed to have estrogenic effects while **Glycyrrhiza, Dioscorea, and Smilax** are observed to have progesterone effects. Most medical practitioners have not had any patients who were totally unresponsive to natural therapeutics for FBD. In the most difficult patients, an iodine supplementation was added to the basic plan of low fat diet plus avoidance of caffeine and vitamin E supplementation.

---

**Botanical Cancer Medicines To Treat Breast Cancer.**

## Dandelion Plant (herb - NOT just the root):-

This is the plant that infests back yards. "Dandelion contains high levels of potassium, is a rich source of iron and vitamins, and, ounce for ounce, contains more carotene than carrots." "Dandelion greens contain 7,000 units of Vitamin A per ounce. It is important to realize that there is always a vitamin A deficiency in a person found to have cancer.

The Chinese have used Dandelion for breast cancer for over a thousand years. Inulin, one of the major chemicals in Dandelion, is currently being studied extensively for its immuno-stimulatory functions.

In testing it against cancer, it has been shown to be active against two tumor systems, by stimulating the actions of the white cells." Actually, the list of cancer-fighting nutrients in dandelions is quite long. "In 1979, Japanese researchers found a dandelion extract - since then patented, which inhibits Erlich ascites cancer cells."

Wild Foods: The Missing Part of Your Diet May Be In Your Own Back Yard:-

Many of those unglamorous "weeds" that you've been poisoning or pulling out of your garden and lawn are some of the world's most well-respected and powerful healing plants? If not, you aren't alone.

Many people don't realize that common ordinary weeds can build and maintain good health. Common weeds that grow by you can boost your immunity, strengthen your liver and help you build strong blood, counter colds and the flu, increase your vitality, and even prevent cancer.

Health-promoting weeds are easy to find, easy to identify, easy to prepare, incredibly abundant, and as delicious as high-priced gourmet goodies. Look or buy one or more of these seven. Burdock, Dandelion,

Honeysuckle, Plantain, Red Clover, Violet, or Yellow Dock. (To the botanist: Arctium lappa, Taraxacum officinale, Plantago majus, Trifolium pratense, Viola odorata, and Rumex crispus.)

How can they change your life? When properly prepared and used, these weeds can boost your immunity, strengthen your liver, renew your energy, and help prevent cancer.

---

**Immune System Boosters:-**

Dandelion and Honeysuckle are particularly good builders of the immune system. (The immune system is a network of cells and cell. products that defends the body against disease-causing organisms such as bacteria, viruses, parasites, and cancer cells.) Dandelion root tincture (20 drops, 2-3 times a day) actually increases the production of interferon, a protein that inhibits viral multiplication and activates T-cells.

Building powerful immunity can help us to remain cancer-free and it provides long-lasting benefits and long life, for relatively little effort.

**Liver Strengtheners:-** The liver is the body's recycling center. This large organ is critical to healthy digestive functioning, utilization of hormones, and removal of chemicals from the body. Dandelion is an outstanding liver strengthener. It is known to protect, heal and tone up the liver, helping to relieve food allergies and aid digestion, as well as repairing damage done by drugs, chemicals, alcohol, and infections such as hepatitis. Burdock, Red Clover, Plantain, and Yellow Dock are also powerful liver strengtheners.

Most experienced healers are unanimous in their agreement that a healthy liver is the basis for a healthy and long life. Perhaps the single most important benefit to be gained from befriending the weeds is the strengthening of your liver function. Dandelion, Yellow Dock, or Burdock roots are used in tinctures (20 drops, 2-3 times a day) or vinegars (1-2large spoonfuls on salad daily); Red Clover is best taken as an infusion; Plantain leaves are eaten in salad or infused in apple cider vinegar.

## Blood Builders:-

Yellow Dock builds strong blood. Strong blood is rich in iron and other minerals needed for health. Strong blood is nutrient-rich- so vital organs get the nourishment they need for optimum functioning. Strong blood helps muscles work well without cramping and aching. Strong blood is low in cholesterol and moves easily through the circulatory system. Strong blood is packed with plenty of energy, for life, for work, and for sex.

Other green allies that build strong blood are Dandelion leaves, Red Clover blossoms, and Plantain leaves (and for strong veins, Burdock root vinegar is a trusted ally). Daily doses of Yellow Dock root vinegar or tincture (5-20drops once or twice a day).

They often increase iron levels in the blood twice as fast as iron supplements. If you wish to avoid alcohol, soak chopped fresh Yellow Dock roots (or any of the other plants mentioned) in vinegar to cover for 6 weeks. I use 1-2 tablespoons a day of the resulting medicinal vinegar to build strong blood.

## Counter Colds and the Flu:-

Throughout the Orient, Honeysuckle flowers are steeped in water and the resulting strong tea, scientifically established as antiseptic, anti-microbial, and anti-infective. They are drunk to ward off colds and the flu. (An injectible form of Honeysuckle is used in Chinese hospitals to counter severe infections.) Red Clover blossoms mixed with ordinary mint and steeped in hot water for several hours is an effective "cold remedy" passed down from Colonial housewives.

## Increase Vitality, Even Prevent Cancer:-

The leaves of Violets and the blossoms of both Honeysuckle and Red Clover are renowned as safe, life-enhancing tonics. In addition to enhancing vitality and rejuvenating fertility, they have proven effectiveness against pre-cancerous conditions.

Red Clover is especially noted for its ability to reverse in situ breast cancers, cervical dysplasias, and pre-cancerous polyps of the colon. Violet, whether drunk in infusion or applied as a poultice, has a reputation as a dissolver of breast lumps and a protector of the lungs, even checking the growth of tumors.

## Anti-cancer Agents:-

The most amazing thing about these seven humble plants is that each of them has been associated with cancer prevention. Plantain is an important Latin-American folk remedy against cancer. Burdock as a specific cure for breast cancer dates back to at least 1887 in the Ukraine.

Around the world, Red Clover is a widely used folk remedy against cancer and is known as "the herb of immortality." Dandelion is known to stop the promotion of oncogenes (when damaged or turned on, an oncogene initiates cancer).Violet slows tumor growth. Honeysuckle is a popular anti-cancer agent in China. Yellow Dock is one of the original plants in the Native American anti-cancer brew now known as Essiac.

As you can see, these seven plants are not just useless weeds.

**Burdock:** Dig first-year roots in Autumn; use mature seeds. Used internally, it resolves chronic skin problems; fresh root binds and removes heavy metals and chemicals. Use daily for six or more weeks; it is not unusual to take burdock regularly for 2 to 3 years. Dried root infusion: 1 to 2 cups. Cooked, dried, or raw root: Eaten freely. Fresh root vinegar: 1-4 tablespoons. Tincture of fresh roots or seeds: 30-250 drops. Infused oil of seeds: As needed on skin or scalp to encourage growth of new hair. Burdock is slow acting but miraculous.

**Dandelion:** Leaves are nourishing, roots are tonifying. Improves outlook, improves digestion and appetite, relieves food allergies. Can use daily for prolonged use. Fresh leaves and flowers: Eaten freely. Cooked greens: 1/2 to 2 cups (125 to 500 ml). Dried root infusion (tea) I to 3 cups (250-750ml).

Tincture of fresh plant, including root: 15-120 drops. Wine of fresh flowers: No more than 6 oz (200 ml). Infused oil of fresh flowers: As needed. Dandelion is a superb ally for liver and breasts. Regular use, internally before meals and externally before sleep helps keep breasts healthy, reverses cancerous changes. Digestion is settled and strengthened a few minutes after taking a dose. Results in breast tissue are slower, taking six weeks or more to become evident.

**Honeysuckle**: One of the most vigorous vines known, Honeysuckle makes an excellent complementary medicine for many Western drugs, moderating or eliminating many of their damaging side effects. The flower buds are harvested in May or June, dried quickly in the sun without turning or handling, infused in water overnight (one ounce dried blossoms to one quart boiling water in a tightly sealed jar steeped for 4-10 hours), and drunk freely.

**Plantain:** Use leaves, harvested any time, or ripe seeds with hulls. Internal use: Seeds are anti-microbial, against thrush. Leaves: Promotes blood clotting, increase in iron, strengthens digestion. Used externally: Leaf poultice or oil reduces cysts, helps prevent cancer, heals skin and connective tissues, stops itching and prevents scars. Daily use: No limit. Raw leaves: 3-20 chopped in salad.

Dried leaf infusion (tea) up to one quart (1 liter). Fresh leaf vinegar: 1-2 tablespoons (15-30ml). Seeds cooked or soaked overnight in cold water: As needed. Fresh leaf oil/ointment or poultice: As needed. Internal response is prompt; noticeable improvement in blood iron is seen in two weeks of daily use. External response is also rapid: Itching ceases, bleeding stops, pain abates, and swelling recedes in minutes. Plantain promotes quick, scarless healing from biopsies, breast surgery and needle sticks. Plantain heals skin and connective tissues, prevents and heals scars.

**Red Clover:** Use the just-opened blossoms with a few leaves clinging. Internally: Alkalinizes, builds blood; helps prevent the recurrence of breast cancer, protects liver and lungs, improves appetite, relieves constipation, eases anxiety; relieves symptoms of premature menopause, increases fertility.

**Externally:** Softens and reduces breast lumps, antifungal. Daily use is without limit. Fresh blossoms: Eaten freely. Infusion (tea) of dried flowers: Up to one quart (1 liter). Tincture/mother tincture of fresh blossoms: 15-100 drops. Fresh flower vinegar: 1-4 tablespoons (15-60ml). Fresh blossom oil/ointment/poultice: As often as needed.

**Note:** Overconsumption of blood-thinning coumarins, which are present only in low amounts in red clover but found in greater amounts in other clovers such as sweet clover, can lead to the breakdown of blood cells and increase risk of hemorrhage. Red clover (legume family) shares with its sisters, soy, lentil and astragalus, the ability to repair damaged DNA, turn off oncogenes, and reverse both pre-cancers and in situ cancers. According to J. Hartwell, author of Plants Used Against Cancer, medical literature has reported and confirmed hundreds of cases of remission of cancer after consistent use of red clover.

**Violet:** Use the leaves, harvested any time, even during flowering. Externally: Eases pain and inflammation, heals mouth sores, softens skin, antifungal. Daily dose: Use without limit, non-toxic. Fresh leaves: In salad, as desired. Dried leaf infusion: Up to one quart (1 liter). Fresh or dried leaf poultice: Continuously. Internal and external use of violet can shrink a breast lump in a month.

**Yellow Dock:** Use roots of a plant at least two years old, dug after autumn frosts, or very early in the spring; leaves, harvested at any time, use ripe seeds. Internally: Roots, builds healthy blood, protects liver, anti-fungal, and checks Candida overgrowth. Used as laxative. As a seed tea, heals mouth sores and checks diarrhea. Externally: Dissolves lumps, anti-tumor and anti-fungal. Can use daily for up to 3 to 12 months. Tincture of fresh roots: 10-60 drops. Fresh root vinegar: 1-2 tablespoons (30 ml). Dried seed tea: No more than one cup (250 ml). Fresh root oil/ointment: Liberally.

### Astragalus:-

This botanical medicine has captured the interest of many conventional doctors because of its ability to reduce the toxic effects of conventional cancer treatment. It appears to protect the liver against the harmful toxic effects of chemotherapy and may be very effective in treating terminally ill cancer patients.

A study in Peking Cancer Institute observed a much higher survival rate among patients with advanced cancers when they were treated with both radiation and astragalus compared to those treated with radiation alone.

## Echinacea:-

This is a well-known immune-enhancing herb. It was found to increase NK (natural killer) cell activity by 90% in patients with inoperable, far-advanced organ cancer when echinacea was combined with a thymus-stimulating agent (thymostimulun).

Also a natural chemical in Echinacea, arabinogalactin, stimulates the tumor-killing activity of macrophages. One of Echinacea's primary roles is to provide protection against infection, a common and sometimes deadly complication in early and advanced-stage cancers.

## Cesium:-

A nonradioactive form of cesium, a rare alkali metal widely distributed in the Earth's crust and listed in the periodic table of elements, it has been used with success as an alternative cancer therapy.

It has been suggested that cesium alkalinizes the body fluids and this, in turn, pushes the normally acidic (low) pH of the cancer cell toward a weakly alkaline (high) pH, promoting the cancer's demise. Thus cesium emerged as a high pH-inducing therapy.

A study reported that cesium chloride, when combined with chelation therapy (a method of binding an organic substance known as a chelating agent to a metallic ion with a positive electric charge [heavy metal] and removing it from the body) and nutritional supplements, led to significant improvement in about half of all "terminal" cancers of the pancreas, colon, gallbladder, liver, breast, prostate, and others most of which had not responded to conventional therapy.

**Shark Cartilage:-**

Another protocol of treatment for cancer is shark cartilage. In 1994, the FDA granted Dr. Charles Simone an Investigational New Drug approval for his treatment of advanced cancers using this substance. Is contains angiogenesis inhibitors, which cut off the blood supply to tumor growth, thereby inhibiting new tumors.

During the clinical trial, he saw 100 patients with various advanced cancers. Some chose only the intensive shark cartilage program and his cancer-fighting plan, and some chose his plan in addition to chemotherapy. Complete remissions occurred in 3 patients.

All the patients in the first group and half of the second experienced better energy levels, less pain, enhanced appetite, and more positive moods. Shark cartilage supplements can be purchased through the mail from any vitamin and supplement store that does mail orders.

Other Botanicals worth looking into for their strong cancer fighting ability are Essiac, Garlic, Grape Seed Extract, Green Tea, Haelan 851, a liquid soybean concentrate, HANSI, a series of homeopathically prepared herbs, and Pau D' Arco, a herbal extract from the bark of South American *Tahebuia* trees, and others mentioned later in this review.

**Green Concentrates:-**

Known as "green drinks" or the "super-vitamin," green concentrates can include chlorella, wheat and barley grass, spirulina, blue-green algae, and alfalfa. One called ProGreens is a dry green powder containing 33 nutritional substances, taken with water or juice, 1-2 times a day.

The benefits, according to ProGreens, include immune support, antioxidant protection, gastrointestinal fortification, energy boosting, and overall nutrient supplementation, all extremely important to fighting cancer and its harmful effects.

ProGreens can be contacted in San Leandro, CA at 510-639-4572. There is also Green Magic from New Spirit Naturals in San Dimas, CA 800-922-2766.

Other Botanicals worth looking into for their strong oral cancer fighting ability are Essiac, Garlic, Grape Seed Extract, Green Tea, Haelan 851, a liquid soybean concentrate, HANSI, a series of homeopathically prepared herbs, and Pau D' Arco, a herbal extract from the bark of South American *Tahebuia* trees, and many others prescribed by an alternative physician.

**An overview of cancer markers:-**

A Cancer "**Marker**" generally refers to any of a variety of standard laboratory blood tests used to measure the level of a protein material or other chemical produced by cancer cells. These numbers become elevated in the presence of a cancer or tumors. X-rays and CT scans are cancer markers also, because they can determine the location of cancer in the body, but the term usually indicates a blood test.

Dr. Jesse Stoff, who is noted along with several other alternative physicians at the end of this review, has observed that cancer markers do not always provide the best indication of the specific character or relative aggressiveness of a cancer.

With breast cancer, for example, there are 4 different cancer markers, but it is rare to find a breast cancer that produces more than 2 or 3 of them. "You can have a huge tumor sitting there and any one of these markers can be well within normal range," Dr. Stoff says.

There is also a less than adequate correlation between cancer markers and the tumor mass. "You can have people with advanced metastatic disease and only moderately elevated levels of cancer markers, and vice versa," Dr. Stoff says.

However, consistent correlations between tumor mass and cancer markers can serve as a rough approximation by how well the battle is going for any one individual, he adds.

When the treatment activates the immune system to respond to the tumor cells, the cancer markers will typically start showing a sudden rise or spike. This is because large amounts of proteins (tumor antigens, or cancer markers) are released as the cancer cells begin to die. "The cancer markers will go through the ceiling at this point,"

Dr. Stoff says. 'One needs to be prepared for this from a psychological point of view." If blood tests are done, cancer patients should realize that the rise will be transient and that it will drop precipitously, usually within 1 to 6 weeks.

During this period, the immune system's scavenging cells, the macrophages, will sweep up the cancer cells' debris. "The take-home lesson is that if you look at cancer markers only, you may get an inaccurate picture of how the cancer is behaving at that time," says Dr. Stoff. "The test should be repeated later on to ensure that the original reading is truly a spike, not an absolute, prolonged rise in the cancer markers."

Third, Dr. Stoff creates a list of all treatment options that may apply or "make biological sense" for this particular cancer. For Dr. Stoff, this may include alternative and conventional treatments as well as combinations of both that might maximize the clinical outcome while minimizing toxic side effects. Many patients treated by alternative physicians have already received extensive conventional treatment and are typically in need of intensive detoxification and immune-enhancing measures.

It is at the point where the cancer patient wants to combine effective strategies for an individual approach to their particular cancer that they should consult an alternative physician clinic, such as the one listed at the bottom of this review, or a qualified holistic health nutritionist. These professionals will use the cancer markers to individually treat and change the treatments appropriately to maximize cancer elimination results.

---

## Dietary Support for Breast Cancer Patients:-

A primarily vegetarian diet is the optimal nutritional strategy for supporting recovery from cancer, determined by objective laboratory tests (blood tests for nutrients, enzymes, hormones, and immune parameters) and subjective measures, such as a person's food tastes and willingness to try a new diet.

Some hormone free chicken and high quality fresh fish can be eaten with (if possible to find) organic vegetables and high quality whole grains, legumes, fruits and nuts. If possible, begin to buy these foods at a local health food market if you are not already doing so.

The digestive capacities of the individual also must be considered, for they play a fundamental role in determining the body's usage of nutrients. Many cancer patients have a weakened digestive system, due to the cancer itself or, more often, the toxic effects of previous treatment by radiation or chemotherapy.

Cooking foods helps because heating the food breaks down the cellulose, making nutrients more available for digestion.

"We usually begin with foods that are basically predigested, such as cooked grains and cooked vegetables, since the cancer patient's enzyme production in the small intestine is typically poor," Dr. Stoff says. "To consume raw vegetables or vegetable juices will cause additional stress because the patient won't digest it or absorb it. To support the digestive system I often recommend an enzyme formula called Absorbaid."

Vegetables can be cooked by quick steaming, being careful not to over-cook, and only whole grains should be cooked and eaten. If one feels they can consume a moderate amount of raw vegetables and especially raw juices, it can make an immediate difference, flooding the body with essential cancer fighting nutrients.

## Enzymes For Digestive Support:-

**Enzymes** are fundamental to all living processes in the body, necessary for every chemical reaction and the normal activity of our organs, tissues, fluids, and cells. There are hundreds of thousands of these Nature's "workers." Enzymes are specialized living proteins that enable your body to digest and assimilate food.

There are special enzymes for digesting proteins, carbohydrates, fats, and plant fibers. Protease digests protein, amylase digests carbohydrates, and lipase digests fats, cellulase for fiber and disaccharidase for sugars.

When a person has cancer, there is a usually a lack of enzymes and/or enzyme dysfunction. This creates an inability for the body to metabolize protein, which may promote cancer.

This inability can be linked to improper amounts of proteolytic (protein-digesting) enzymes such as pepsin from the stomach and proteases from the pancreas which, along with hydrochloric acid (HCI) in the stomach, which are the body's first defense against cancer. Enzyme therapy can is an important step in restoring health and well-being by helping to remedy digestive dysfunction.

Both plant-derived enzymes and animal-derived pancreatic enzymes are used in enzyme therapy. One should seek to supplement with a whole food supplement that provides both nutrition and enzymes.

---

**Nutritionals to Add to fight Breast Cancer:-**

This is a general overview of nutritionals, and there are many more. They idea is to begin to supplement with these and others prescribed by a qualified nutritionist so that the body can get a much needed boost in fighting cancer.

One reason a cancer patient may feel so ill during conventional treatments is that the accumulation of the cancer cells' cellular debris is built up in the body in high levels. If the body does not eliminate these toxins, a patient can feel sick, nauseous, and achy, have headaches, and flu-like symptoms.

The only way to clear this up is through adequate nutrition and proper elimination. One must make sure to intake all the nutrients below, drink plenty of water, and look into certain types of toxicity-reducing enemas given by a qualified alternative practitioner.

**Acidophilus:-**
A generic term for the **Lactobacilli**, "**friendly bacteria**" naturally inhabits

the healthy intestine. It is very important to cancer therapy for these reasons: It exerts direct activity against cancers, it prevents cancer by detoxifying and preventing the formation of carcinogenic chemicals, reduces cholesterol which indirectly aids cancer resistance, helps produce important B vitamins, and curbs or destroys potentially pathogenic bacteria and hostile yeasts such as Candida albicans, resulting in freeing the immune system to fight cancer cells, and of great importance, through producing lactic acid, preserve and enhance the digestibility of foods which are fermented with them, such as soy products, sauerkraut, pickles and more.

**L. acidophilus** can significantly lower the cancer-triggering activity of compounds in the feces of persons who eat meat.

### Amino Acids:-
These create protein, and are also important to cancer therapy. Humans make 12 of these, but must ingest 8 of the essential ones. Some, our body makes under stress situations, but cannot make enough and it will benefit the body greatly to supplement with one such as glutamine. A test called a fasting plasma sample determines amino acid deficiencies, and if any our lacking, they can be added.

Particular **amino acids** beneficial in cancer treatment are L-arginine, which enhances NK cells, cytoxic T cells and others, Methionine, which should be taken with choline, Cysteine, which assists in detoxification and reduces side effects of chemotherapy and radiation.

### Beta Carotene:-
This is converted to vitamin A when the body needs it, is an antioxidant and immune-enhancing supplement that has properties not found in vitamin A.

### Calcium:-
Taken with magnesium is very important, particularly for bone metastasis

or bone cancers. There is a study that found that calcium deficiency was associated with a higher risk of colorectal cancer. Humans rarely get enough calcium into their diet, and supplementing with it should be for everyone.

### Chromium:-
Taken as either chromium picolinate or chromium polynicotinate, this may help people regain normal thyroid function, which can then bolster thyroid function. It also helps regulate blood sugar levels and this can substantially improve immune function and cancer resistance. Refined foods such as white sugar and flour are nutritionally defunct of chromium, unlike whole grains, and these substances can also deplete the body of chromium.

### Coenzyme Q10 (COQ10)]:-
Also known as ubiquinone, it is essential for generating energy in living things that use oxygen. The body produces some coQ10, but less with aging, and eating foods that contain it is very important, such as fish, especially sardines, soybean and grape seed oils, sesame seeds, pistachios, walnuts, and spinach.

When combines with vitamin E, selenium, and beta-carotene, coQ10 can significantly reduce free-radical damage in the liver, kidney and heart tissues. Some recent findings show that supplementation with coQ10 can cause complete regression of tumors in advanced breast cancer.

### Copper:-
A trace element that is essential to proper functioning of a many immune cell types, which fight and defend against cancer. It is vital to healing processes, excretion of toxins, forming red blood cells, and maintaining connective tissues. It is important to resist infections and also affects inflammation.

### Eicosapentenoic Acid (EPA Fish Oils) Essential Fatty Acids:-

These are required for proper metabolism. They include linoleic and alpha linolenic acid and are found in flaxseed oil, certain seeds, nuts and vegetables. They are important in reducing heart disease and prevention and treatment of various cancers. It is very important to assist they body to fight cancer with the supplement flaxseed oil, which exerts a strong anticancer effect, and animal studies show 50% reductions in tumor size after 1-2 months of supplementation.

**Botanicals That Fortify The Immune System:-**

There are a wide range of botanicals, and we will evaluate two that are noted to be indispensable to effective cancer treatment. Iscador (known as European mistletoe or Viscum album) and Larix (or Arabinogalactan). These botanicals work in a complementary fashion to support the body's anticancer defenses.

**Iscador**-From the holistic point of view, Iscador's unique therapeutic value, its specific effect on tumors, lies in its ability to counteract the disorderly spread of the carcinoma.

According to Hans Richard Heiligtag, M.D., this action results from mistletoe's "strict formative force which expresses itself in its regular rhythmical growth, and on the other hand in its special relation to light and warmth, which enables it to blossom in wintertime. These three factors enable mistletoe to be a cancer remedy.

In other words, the strong force counteracts the revolt of the forces, which characterize the malignant cell. At the same time, the ability to counteract the cold of wintertime carries over into mistletoe's ability to counteract the "coldness" that characterizes the cancer-ridden body-cancer patients often complain of feeling cold, but their bodies become warmer after treatment with mistletoe.

Typically, European doctors using Iscador administer the first series of injections to observe any undesirable reactions. The medicine is injected (subcutaneous, as a serum) in the morning, several times per week. Iscador can be taken orally, either as a tincture or in homeopathic form, but only if the immune system is already 'somewhat responsive.' If one's immune system is weak or severely compromised then the injection is recommended. "

The strength that we use for injecting Iscador depends on the energy reserves of the patient and how much immune reserve they have left," says Stoff. "However, all the injections are low potency."

**Larix-Larch Arabinogalactan Powder, or Ara-6:-** A sweet-tasting medicinal powder highly concentrated in complex carbohydrates or polysaccharides (long-chain sugars) derived from the Western Larch tree (Larix occidentalis). A special property it has is its capacity for stimulating the activity of various types of immune cells. Ara-6 also dissolves in water easily and maintains its chemical stability over a wide range of concentrations, pH, and temperature changes.

Definitive results with Larix have been seen in terms of increasing natural killer (NK) cell activity. "We know that NK activity can help a person with cancer, particularly when trying to prevent new tumors or micrometastases. "Larix seems to stimulate NK activity quite well while also helping to raise the individual's energy level," states Dr Stoff. Ara-6 also has the ability to stimulate the activity of macrophages, another major part of the body's anticancer defenses, which may be just as significant as its positive effect on NK activity.

Biochemists have determined that a sugar component of Larix may stimulate NK activity in a manner similar to the sugar component of Viscum album (mistletoe).' The combination of these substances could therefore have an additive effect in terms of activating anticancer defenses. Dr. Stoff recommends taking a teaspoon in a glass of vegetable juice or water times a day. Typically people who take Ara-6 are advised to take supplemental vitamin C at the same time because it can enhance the effectiveness of Ara-6. Both of these botanicals may be acquired and administered by a qualified alternative physician of nutritionalist.

## The Importance of Detoxification in a Cancer Reversal Program:-

Most alternative medicine doctors and holistic practitioners agree that too many toxins in the body produce illness. Signs and symptoms of the toxic body can include being overweight, bloating and intestinal gas, insomnia, nausea, bad breath, asthma, constipation, tension, headaches, depression, stress, allergies, weakness, intense menstrual discomforts and problems, and many others.

Cancer patients wishing to get a head start on eliminating cancer from their body must seek a form of detoxification, which will maximize results of eliminating cancer from the body and if one is going through conventional treatment, a detoxifying program will maximize the results as well

Many cancer patients who seek alternative treatments have already had conventional treatment and are already nutritionally depleted and overloaded with toxins. If this were the case, it would be highly dangerous to attempt a strong detoxification program. It is a delicate balance in these cases where the liver's functioning should be stimulated in a gentle and gradual way while supporting the immune system.

A patient should try to ingest foods and herbs to reduce stress on a toxic organ or body region. In the case of an overburdened liver, a botanical medicine such as Essiac is good to ingest, which has "an affinity for the liver and doesn't stress the kidneys," states Dr. Stoff.

Also good to take is **silymarin** (milk over thistle). "This herb is valuable in helping cancer patients recover from the toxic effects of chemotherapy or heavy drug use in general. No other single herb seems to have as much detoxifying, liver-regenerating power."

Some people specify juicing and ingesting nothing but raw juice for detoxification and intense immune boosting. It is not always recommended that one drink large amounts of raw juices such as carrot juice at first, as is sometimes recommended for cancer patients, because the liver generally cannot fully convert the beta carotene in carrots to vitamin A.

Small amounts, sometimes diluted with two part pure water (two parts carrot juice) is desirable in cases where the liver is not over- burdened.

The effort alone to digest properly large amounts of raw juice can place an additional stress on the body. An overly toxic liver can be relieved through simple dietary changes such as avoiding oils and high-fat foods and emphasizing raw leafy greens and brightly colored vegetables.

Once steps have been taken to relieve a toxic liver and one is feeling fairly well, a regimen of drinking raw juices, especially carrot and wheat grass juice can help the body fight cancer cells and other invading problems such as viruses.

A toxic kidney is another condition commonly seen among cancer patients, particularly in those who have received extensive conventional treatments. If the kidneys are not functioning well, patient should be careful with supplements, such as large amounts of amino acids, minerals, and high-dose vitamin C. The reason for this is that these nutrients are all water-soluble and pass through the kidney to be eliminated through urination. Instead, one would want to take these slowly, as healing is under way and under the supervision a qualified nutritionist.

In general, when the elimination system is in a toxic and not functioning well, the reason for the poor response must be determined. A toxic colon or kidney means there are elevated creatinine, constipation, gas, bloating, cramps, and often a skin rash.

A heavy meat-eating diet is the number one cause particularly when coupled with a sedentary lifestyle. Starting a regular exercise program (one tailored to the specific needs of the individual and reviewed by their physician) and abstaining from eating lots of meat can make an immediate difference.

The colon can sometimes be stimulated to work better by checking out some substances that a nutritionist might recommend. These could include **Epsom salts**, taken orally, Chinese herbs (such as San She Dan), and special fiber supplements all individually determined with the help of a nutritionist, to stimulate the colon, and help it work better. There are several detoxification packages that one can purchase also.

Working from below, the use a coffee enema is very effective and can be administered by a holistic health practitioner specializing in colonic irrigation therapy. This is the only detoxifying technique some physicians working alternatively use on a routine basis with cancer patients. It is used primarily to stimulate liver detoxification.

Let's see how **Milk thistle** is increasingly used to promote general health and efficient detoxification, to protect against environmental pollutants and to **reduce the toxic side effects of drugs used in chemotherapy.**

Traditionally considered a liver tonic, milk thistle is used in Europe for chronic hepatitis and cirrhosis (liver malfunction). Clinical studies suggest that standardized milk thistle seed extract may also protect against liver damage from exposure to hazardous chemicals.

**RECENT FINDINGS:-** An article published in the 2001 issue of Drugs concluded that silymarin significantly reduced liver-related deaths from cirrhosis. Silymarin also reduced the amount of insulin required by people suffering from cirrhosis-related diabetes.

Preliminary studies suggest that milk thistle may have anticancer effects. This is attributed to the strong antioxidant action of silymarin.

Researchers are also examining whether milk thistle may both prevent the toxic side effects of some cancer treatments (cyclosporine and cisplatin) and **enhance the cancer-fighting** ability of other medications.

**POSSIBLE SIDE EFFECTS:** Side effects with milk thistle are very rare; however, mild laxative effects and possible allergic reactions — primarily skin rashes — have occasionally been reported.

---

## Pharmaceuticals Substances for Treating Cancer:-

## Alkylglycerols (Shark Liver Oil):-

A group of compounds called alkylglycerols (pronounced all-kill-gliss-ser-alls) can bolster anticancer defenses and protect the body against the harmful effects of radiation-induced injury." The richest source of these special fats (also called "ether lipids" or "alkyllyso phospholipids") is shark liver oil, but these fats' are found to a lesser extent in mother's milk, which contains 10 times more alkylglycerols than cow's milk.

Animal studies have indicated that alkylglycerols have anti-tumor activity, probably mediated through certain immune cells (macrophages) in the form of direct and selective destruction to cancer cells. Cell culture studies have shown that alkylglycerols are 'selectively toxic against cancer cells" and this "selection" seems to be affected by the cholesterol concentration of the cancer cell; as the cholesterol level drops, the cancer cells die more rapidly.

Extracts of shark liver oil may help people tolerate both chemotherapy and radiation. The administration of alkylglycerols prior to radiation treatment was found to cause advanced tumors to regress toward less advanced stages; alkylglycerols also caused reversal of tumor growth in animal studies.

A possible explanation for these findings is that this substance can inhibit a variety of tumor-promoting substances, including the "bad" eicosanoids and platelet-activating factor (PAF). One potential area of concern, however, is contamination of shark liver oil by ocean pollutants.

No published research that is known of has yet neither addressed this issue nor have the potential toxicities at normal doses been adequately studied.

Scientists at Johns Hopkins University School of medicine found that a synthetic form of squalamine, originally derived from shark liver, is effective in controlling the growth of brain tumors in rats and in extending their lives. The substance suppresses the formation of new blood vessels in the tumor, thus preventing it from growing, reports the New York Times (May 1, 1996).

With their toothsome maws and machine-like killing efficiency, the primitive creatures known as sharks have long inspired fear and commanded respect. But does this ancient family of boneless fish harbor a secret weapon against some of the most dreaded cancers afflicting humans?

Centuries ago, Scandinavian practitioners of folk medicine adopted the habit of consuming shark liver oil as a general health tonic. In recent decades, scientists have observed that tumors are remarkably rare in sharks, and that these predatory fish are notoriously resistant to infections.' This amazing imperviousness to disease doubtless inspired the folk remedy.

Admittedly, fighting disease with shark oil sounds far-fetched. The very notion evokes unsavory images of cure-all tonics and unscrupulous charlatans from centuries past. But in 1952, Dr. Astrid Brohult stumbled upon remarkable proof that shark oil actually works.

The fascinating story of her discovery, related by some of her colleagues in the book Shark Liver Oil: Natures Amazing Healer, provides a glimpse at the happy serendipity that occasionally results when science and intuition mix.

Dr. Brohult was a young Swedish oncologist working with leukemia patients in a children's hospital. Leukemia is a potentially deadly cancer that affects white blood cells, or leukocytes, which are the immune system's front-line defensive players, manufactured in the bone marrow. When leukemia strikes, leukocyte production runs amok.

To stop the disease, patients are exposed to enough radiation to kill the cells in the bone marrow that give rise to both red and white blood cells. This drastic treatment is usually effective, but occasionally may be worse than the disease itself.

With fewer red blood cells to carry oxygen and remove wastes, and few leukocytes left to fight infection and marshal other defenses, patients are rendered weak, deathly ill, and prone to infection.

In an effort to stimulate her patients' bone marrow to resume normal function, Dr. Brohult administered calve's marrow to the children in her care. She was operating on little more than a hunch. Parents in Scandinavia have long served bone marrow soup to their children in winter, in the belief that it builds up a person's strength.

---

## Antineoplastons:-

Beginning in the 1960's, Stanislaw Burzynski, M.D., isolated several peptides (chains of amino acids, the building blocks of protein) from human urine and found them to be effective in controlling the growth of certain types of cancer. Dr. Burzynski originally identified and isolated from the urine of healthy humans 5 different antineoplastons (meaning substances that work against [anti] a neoplasm [an abnormal growth of new tissue, such as a tumor]).

He determined that these molecules have a strong anticancer effect at a genetic level: specifically, they appear to stimulate the activity of "tumor suppressor genes," genes that literally turn off the activity of certain oncogenes (genes that promote tumor growth). By this action, antineoplastons can actually stop cells from multiplying out of control, eventually producing a tumor mass, said Dr. Burzynski. It is almost as if cancer results from a deficiency of antineoplastons.

Dr. Burzynski has successfully used antineoplastons, which he produces himself in an FDA-approved manufacturing facility in his Houston, Texas', clinic. Currently, he has 65 different treatment protocols using 2 antineoplaston formulas. The protocols differ according to type and size of tumor, although best results appear to come from treating brain tumors, metastatic breast cancer, and non-Hodgkin's lymphoma.

As part of a study, he used antineoplastons to treat 20 patients who had advanced-stage astrocytoma, a particularly fast-growing type of brain tumor that tends to occur in young children. Nearly 80% of them responded favorably, and a number of them were tumor free 4 years later. At the Ninth International Symposium on Future Trends in Chemotherapy in March 1990, Dr. Dvorit Samid stated, "Antineoplaston AS2-1 profoundly inhibits oncogene expression and the proliferation of malignant cells without exhibiting any toxicity toward normal cells. 'Based on clinical results of 7 studies presented at the conference, Dr. Samid concluded: "Antineoplaston therapy restores to the body those natural compounds that have anticancer activity. Because they are natural compounds, the body tolerates them well, and therefore we minimize the problem of adverse effects.

**Antineoplastons** could be a very **valuable, effective, and safe approach to cancer therapy.** The inhibitory effect of Antineoplaston A-10 was tested on the growth curve of **human breast cancer (R-27)** serially transplanted to athymic mice and on the cell growth of human hepatocellular carcinomas (KMCH-1, KYN-1, KIM-1).

Approximately 1.25% of Antineoplaston A-10 in the regular mouse diet (CE2) inhibited the growth curve significantly after 35 days treatment ($p<0.05$). Seventy milligrams of daily intraperitoneal administration of Antineoplaston A-10 Injection also inhibited the growth curve of R-27 after 52 days treatment ($p<0.01$).

Histological study of tumor showed no essential difference in structure but significant decrease in number of mitoses in the Antineoplaston A-10 treated groups. The cell growth of human hepatocellular carcinoma cell lines KMCH-1, KYN-1 and KIM-1 was inhibited by Antineoplaston A-10 Injection dose dependently.

More evidence that Antineoplaston A-10 has been shown to have negligible toxicity in acute and chronic studies in animals.

Antineoplastons did not exhibit any mutagenic activity in the standardized Ames test. Antineoplaston A-10 is quite insoluble in water and partly hydrolyzed in pancreatic juice to phenylacetylglutamine and phenylacetylisoglutamine in the ratio of 4:1.

The sodium salt of phenylacetylglutamine and phenylatylisoglutamine was formulated as Antineoplaston A-10 Injection because both these two degradation products were found to have inhibitory effect on neoplastic cell growth in tissue culture study. Although Burzynski reported antitumor effects of both oral and injectable formulations of Antineoplaston A-10 in clinical studies (Burzynski et al. 1984, 1986), an antitumor effect of this substance has never been reported in an animal model.

Thus, we designed animal experiments to test for an antitumor effect of Antineoplaston A-10 on human breast cancer (R-27) transplanted to athymic m ice (Nawata et al. 1981) as well as for an inhibitory effect on human hepatocellular carcinoma cell lines (KlM-1, KYN-1, KMCH-1).

The discrepancy between animal and clinical results regarding antitumor effect of oral formula and injection formula of Antineoplaston A-10 could be at least partly explained as due to the dose of Antineoplaston A-10 administered and maintained.

Because the effect of Antineoplaston A-10 is cytostatic, longer and careful observation is required to evaluate the antitumor effect of the agent especially in animals. The great potential of this agent in inducing change in protein synthesis by the tumor cells should be investigated from the point of view of application for the cancer chemotherapy.

---

**Carnivora:-**
This extract of the meat-eating plant Venus' flytrap (Dinoea muscipula) was introduced into cancer therapy by German oncologist Helmet Keller, medical director of the Chronic Disease Control and Treatment Center in Bad Steven, Germany. Dr. Keller has conducted extensive studies of the intravenous delivery of Carnivora as used in German cancer clinics.

The medicine contains one-third pressed Venus flytrap juice, one-third alcohol, and one-third purified water. Dr. Keller has treated over 2,000 cancer patients with Camivora, so named in honor of the plant's well-known insect-eating ability.

One of the active ingredients appears to be a chemical called plumbagin which has anticancer properties;" when topically applied, it can lead to a total reversal of skin cancer."

Dr. Keller's laboratory studies indicate that Camivora directly inhibits the metabolic activity of cancer cells. In a clinical study of 210 cancer patients for whom conventional treatments had failed, each received 50-60 drops of Camivora orally 5 times a day plus one intravenous infusion daily.

The results were excellent: 16% of patients showed tumor remission and 40% had no further tumor progression; in the remaining 44% no improvement was noted, although about one-quarter of these patients experienced a palliative effect.

This means they felt a decrease in subjective complaints and pain and an increase in appetite, vitality, and positive attitude, according to Dr. Keller. The study showed that more than half, or 56%, experienced either a tumor remission or their cancer development became stable and did not worsen.

**Camivora is an immunomodulator,** which means it stimulates the activity of T helper cells. This in turn enables the body to wage a more vigorous defense against the illness, explains Dr. Keller. Carnivore appears to target tumor cells and bolster the immune system.

After the intravenous program is completed, intramuscular injections may be carried out several times a week until the treatment program is finished.

People should not attempt to produce their own Camivora, however, since it first must be purified of naturally occurring plant toxins that would otherwise cause fevers and other adverse reactions. Instead, they should contact one of the alternative physicians listed below or a qualified nutritionist for more information.

Carnivora supplies essential nutrients to the immune system allowing it to operate at high efficiency, by allowing it to operate at maximum efficiency.

In addition, it mimics the activities of the immune system itself in destroying defective or so-called primitive cells from a wide variety of pathogens (viruses and bacteria). Many laboratory studies worldwide have demonstrated its effectiveness against cancer and aids. Since 1981, over 2000 patients have been treated with Carnivora, including President Ronald Reagan.

### Bovine Cartilage:-

In 1954, John F. Prudden, M.D., discovered that bovine cartilage had a remarkable ability to help wounds heal faster. Today, bovine tracheal cartilage is one of the few substances proven to accelerate wound healing, which is why most surgical textbooks mention it.

But Dr. Prudden became deeply intrigued with the wider therapeutic potential of this obscure substance. He was able to observe it dramatically shrink a breast tumor and reduce the malignant ulceration of the chest wall of a desperate patient, and he was convinced.

The development of **new blood vessels** (angiogenesis) is a prerequisite for tumor growth, yet this process can be **stopped by cartilage** from either cows or sharks.

Bovine tracheal cartilage (BTC) causes a general activation of the body's anticancer defenses and has demonstrated effectiveness against cancers of the ovary, pancreas, colon, and testes; a BTC extract inhibited the growth of tumor cell lines from 22 Patients with various cancers.

Since 1972, Dr. Pradden has used BTC to successfully treat many cases of advanced cancer; the partial and complete response rate, taken overall, is approximately 30% within a 7-month treatment period.

In a now classic study released in 1985, Dr. Pradden reported on the results of a trial with 31 cancer patients all of whom had failed to respond to conventional therapies or had a cancer that was not treatable at all. After starting a regimen of cartilage- typically 9 g daily, taken orally in 3 - gram installments 3 times daily, 90% of the patients had a partial or complete response.

Dr. Prudden also reports success in causing a large rectal tumor to disappear, leaving the patient cancer free for 18 years after treatment.

Bovine cartilage produced a complete healing of breast cancer after all other therapies had failed; this patient remained free of cancer for IO years until her death from other causes.

A man with prostatic cancer that had spread to the bones had a complete remission. An elderly woman, aged 79, with kidney cancer that had spread to her lungs and liver, survived 4 years with much improved conditions.

Strictly speaking it is not a cure because patients who respond to it must continue taking it at the rate of 9 mg. daily for the rest of their lives to avoid a possible remission. It also takes up to 4 months for the initial positive effects to show up in the system, Dr. Prudden advises. In more than 2 5 years, he has never observed any toxic side effects from using bovine cartilage, even with doses 3 times as high as the therapeutic dose.

Bovine cartilage also contains large sugar molecules called mucopolysaccharides that appear to block cell division in the cancerous cells. If the cells cannot divide, they cannot multiply, which means the **cancer doesn't spread**.

For the therapeutic dose needed, bovine cartilage if 4 times less expensive than shark cartilage and it takes approximately 70 g of shark cartilage to get healing results in contrast to 9 grams of bovine cartilage.

Other alternative pharmacological substances worth checking into which are relatively unknown except to alternative cancer physicians are Hydrazine Sulfate, a synthetic chemical which inhibits the loss of protein or body mass caused by cancer; Indocin (Indomethancin) which is a member of the family of nonsteroidal medications and growing research indicates that indocin may be effective against various cancers; Mellitin, derived from the stinger of honeybees, Nucleic Acids (2LC1 and 2 LCL1), which are two homeopathic blends that have been shown to be effective in advanced cancers; and 714X, a compound consisting of nitrogen-rich camphor and organic salts that seem effective against many forms of cancer. All of these must be taken under the supervision of a physician or qualified nutritionist.

Dr. Prudden has published a 31 patient case series in which he records some remarkable remissions in a wide variety of intractable malignancies including **Pancreatic Cancer, Metastatic Breast Cancer, and Glioblastoma Multiforme.**

Some of these patients had been followed for more than five years at the time the case series was published in 1985. According to the National Cancer Institute, Bovine Cartilage, a type of tough, flexible connective tissue, has been studied and shown to "have some value" in cancer therapy.

As indicated, various preparations of cartilage from sharks have been studied in the laboratory and in animals for their ability to **kill cancer cells,** stimulate the immune system, and block formation of new blood vessels feeding cancer cells.

Nevertheless, NCI's official public position remains that scientific evidence to date has not proven cartilage to be an effective treatment for cancer. Several formal human clinical trials at NCI are now underway.

**Alternative Clinical Approaches:-**
**Heat Therapy**:- A clinical process called **hyperthermia**, which is the raising of the body's temperature to destroy abnormal cells. It is also called **cauterization** or **electrodiathermy**.

It is another detoxification technique used with some success as part of **an alternative cancer treatment program**.

For example, heat can be localized with the help of medical devices that direct microwaves to the tumor, raising the temperature of the tumor itself to 42' C or 43' C (107.6' F to 109.4' F); this procedure is particularly effective in controlling superficial tumors located on or near the skin.

Conventional doctors have used this approach, known by them as **diathermy** (DYE-a-ther-mee), to lower the effective dosage range of radiation treatment. In the process, patients can reduce or even eliminate the need for radiation therapy. "Only a relatively small rise in body temperature can make a huge difference," says Robert Atkins, M.D., who includes it in his cancer protocols.

Though the principle sounds simple, the technique is far more complicated, thanks to the body's ability to regulate its internal temperature.

As any sauna enthusiast will attest, the human body likes heat only to a point. When the body temperature rises, blood flow increases to dissipate the excess heat.

One way to circumvent the body's ability to regulate its temperature is to apply the heat locally, targeting a specific tumor. This can be done with the use of microwave's and ultrasound, which can be directed at parts of the body with great precision.

Ultrasound causes an increase in body temperature as a result of friction produced at the molecular level as the high-energy sound waves strike different body tissues. (For whole-body or large-area treatments, multiple ultrasound applicators may be used.) Radiant heating devices produce infrared heat that is applied to the body.

Extracorporeal heating involves removing blood from the body (via plastic tubes placed into the veins), heating it, and returning it to the body at a higher temperature.

Normally, the cancer cells, enabling some to survive, repair part of the damage caused by radiation; however, heat foils this self-repairability.

Taken together, these facts tend to make tumors more vulnerable to heat treatment than normal tissue.

At the Duke Hyperthermia Program of the Duke University Medical Center in Durham, North Carolina, considerable success has been reported in using hyperthermia to treat soft-tissue sarcomas and often-deadly recurrences of breast cancer.

One recent study found that radiation combined with hyperthermia was 30% more effective against breast cancer than radiation treatment alone. Tumors located near the surface of the body appear to be more amenable to treatment than deep-tissue tumors. "I try never to use radiation treatment - which is even more dangerous than most forms of chemotherapy-without also using hyperthermia," says Dr. Atkins. "Thanks to hyperthermia, we can shrink tumors with far less radiation today to get the same therapeutic outcome in cancer patients, and our patients' immune systems and overall health are faring much better as a result."

**Hyperthermia** is now approved in the U.S. for treatment of breast cancer recurrence, and it is covered by insurance. This is how heat therapy works: Heat results when atoms and molecules vibrate and move around at a higher rate or frequency.

The body uses its own internally generated heat to protect itself from viruses, bacteria, and other harmful substances. A fever is the body's highly evolved attempt to destroy invading organisms and to sweat impurities out through the skin. Fever is an effective natural process of curing disease and restoring health; heat therapy, or hyperthermia, represents a way to create fever to call out this natural healing process.

Cancer cells are more heat sensitive than normal tissues and are more easily killed by heating. Localizing the heat is important, since one cannot raise the whole-body temperature to 42' C or 43' C without lethal consequences.

Another strategy is to raise the whole-body temperature in a more moderate way, from 3 7' C to 40' C (98.6' F to 104' E). Using whole-body wet wraps, saunas, and hot baths may perform this. When used in combination with taking ginseng or other substances that increase the effect of heat, it can be of value in cancer treatment.

One may also take a hot bath with a cup of Epsom salts and a cup of baking soda mixed into the bath water, which can heat the body to a moderate degree and provide a gentle detoxifying effect.

One substance that may be combined with hyperthermia to enhance its effectiveness is the bioflavonoid quercetin. This bioflavonoid helps stop histamine release. Quercetin can inhibit the synthesis of proteins (heat shock proteins) that help tumors resist heat stress; also quercetin inhibits the transport of lactic acid out of cancer cells. By doing this, it lowers the pH inside the cancer cell and reduces the likelihood that tumor cells will proliferate or metastasize.

Thus, the anticancer effect of quercetin in the context of hyperthermia is twofold: it makes the inside of cancer cells more acidic (lowers the intracellular pH, which helps kill the cell) and makes the cancer cells more vulnerable to the effects of heat. Dr. Stoff's typical dosage is 1000-1500 mg taken 3 times daily.

Only recently has conventional medicine caught up with this practice and begun to incorporate hyperthermia in the orthodox treatment protocols for cancer.

**Exercise:-**To give the detoxification systems an added boost, it is frequently advised patients to engage in regular stress-free physical activities such as walking, jogging, cycling, or swimming.

Gentle games with constant movement such as volleyball and basketball can help stimulate the lymphatic system and overall metabolism, thereby aiding detoxification.

If one has access to a yoga class, this can be of invaluable assistance in stimulating immunity and lowering stress by movement and heating of the body without hard impact.

Exercise speeds up the neutralization and removal of poisons from the body's cells and tissues through sweating and increased urination and stimulate the activity of natural killer cells and other components of the body's anticancer defenses.

When the bodies temperature rises during exercise there tends to be an increase in the production of pyrogen, a substance that enhances the function of white blood cells and thus immune function.

However, excessive exercise can be detrimental. Dr. Stoff cautions that it can produce an excess of free radicals and lactic acid, both of which tend to promote cancer.

Patients should become involved in an exercise program in a gradual and sensitive manner, respecting their abilities and attitudes. "A fundamentalist Christian will often walk out of your office if you suggest they practice yoga," Dr. Stoff says. "It's important to understand where a person is coming from in their beliefs and to support them; otherwise your recommendations will likely fall on deaf ears."

---

**Cancer and AIDS Cured by Hyper-Oxygenation:-**Several dozen AIDS patients have not only reversed their death sentences, but are now back at work, **completely free of the disease**.

They destroyed the virus in their blood by hyper-oxygenation, known in various forms as oxygen therapy, bio-oxidative therapy or auto-hemotherapy. This is a simple, inexpensive and very broadspectrum healing process that many feel could force a complete overhaul of the medical industry. The two basic types of oxygen therapy are ozone blood infusion, and absorption of oxygen water (hydrogen peroxide) at very low concentrations.

It turns out that the AIDS virus cannot tolerate high oxygen levels in its victims' blood. Not only that, every other disease organism tested so far apparently has the same weakness. Even **cancer growths contract and disappear** when the oxygen saturation is sufficiently increased in the fluids surrounding them, since they are **anaerobic.** *Anaerobic* means "living in the absence of air", as opposed to aerobic which means "living in the presence of air."

AIDS, herpes, hepatitis, Epstein Barr, cytomegalovirus and other lipid-envelope virus are readily destroyed by hyper-oxygenating the patient's blood with ozone. This was demonstrated by, among others, Dr. Horst Kief in Bad Hersfeld, West Germany.

Dr. Kiefhas already cured a number of AIDS victims by drawing blood, infusing it with ozone and returning it to the patient, at regular intervals until all the virus is gone. (He can be reached through Biozon Ozon-Technik GmbH, An Der Haune #10, Bad Hersfeld, D-6430, Federal Republic of Germany.)

Dr. S. Rilling of Stuttgart and Dr. Renate Viebahn of Iffezheim are among the growing number of physicians who have obtained similar results with their patients. They are with Arztlich Gesellschaft fur Ozontherapie and JrJ Hansler GmbH, respectively.

**Cancer Cured by Hyper-Oxygenation:-**AIDS, herpes, hepatitis, Epstein Barr, cytomegalovirus and other **lipid-envelope virus** are readily destroyed by hyper-oxygenating the patient's blood with ozone.

**Magnetic Field Therapy:-**The use of magnets and electrical devices to generate controlled magnetic fields has many medical applications and has proven to be one of the most effective means available for diagnosing human illness and disease.

Clinical evidence shows that cancers, subjected to a negative magnetic field, can start to reverse as the magnetic energy helps restore oxygen levels and reduce acidity.

Electromagnetic energy is an integral part of the human body. The world is surrounded by magnetic fields: some are generated by the Earth's magnetism; others are generated by solar storms and changes in the weather. Magnetic fields are also created by everyday electrical devices: motors, televisions, office equipment, computers, electrically heated water beds, electric blankets, microwave ovens, the electrical wiring in homes, and the Power lines that supply them.

The human body produces subtle magnetic fields that are generated by the chemical reactions within the cells and the ionic currents of the nervous system. The catalytic reactions of enzymes are all driven by magnetic fields and produce magnetic fields themselves."

Recently, scientists have discovered that external magnetic fields can affect the body's functioning in both positive and negative ways, and this observation has led to the development of magnetic field therapy.

The use of magnets and electrical devices to generate controlled magnetic fields has many medical applications and has proven to be one of the most effective means available for diagnosing human illness and disease. In addition to its diagnostic power, magnetic field therapy can be used to treat physical and emotional disorders.

Magnets and electromagnetic therapy devices are now being used to relieve symptoms and reverse degenerative diseases, eliminate pain, facilitate the healing of broken bones, counter the effects of stress, and address the reversal of cancer.

In 1974, researcher Albert Roy Davis noted that positive and negative magnetic energies have different effects upon the biological systems of animals and humans. He found that magnets could be used to arrest and kill cancer cells in animals, and could also be used in the treatment of arthritis, glaucoma, infertility, and diseases related to aging.

Davis concluded that negative polarity magnetic fields have a beneficial effect on living organisms, whereas positive polarity magnetic fields have a stressful effect.

In tests to evaluate the risk to cancer patients of exposure to magnetic fields, tissue cultures were exposed to a positive magnetic field for a prolonged period. The cancer grew. With prolonged exposure to a negative magnetic field, the cancer receded.

**Magnetic Field Therapy as a Primary or Adjunctive Cancer Treatment:-**According to Wolfgang Ludwig, So.D. Ph.D., Director of the Institute for Biophysics in Horn, Germany, "Magnetic field therapy is a method that penetrates the whole human body and can treat every organ without chemical side effects."

At Dr. Ludwig's Institute for Biophysics, magnetic field therapy has been effective in the treatment of cancer. Robert Becker, M.D., an orthopedic surgeon and prime researcher of magnetic energy, found that weak electric currents promote the healing of broken bones.

Dr. Becker also brought national attention to the fact that electromagnetic interference from power lines and home appliances can pose a serious hazard to human health. "The scientific evidence leads to only one conclusion: The exposure of living organisms to abnormal electromagnetic fields results in significant abnormalities in physiology and function."

**With Magnetic Field Therapy, Energy Changes At The Cellular Level:-** There are numerous forms of magnetic field therapy, including static field magnets and pulsating magnetic fields generated by electrical devices. The magnetic fields produced by magnets or electromagnetic generating devices are able to penetrate the human body and therapeutically affect the functioning of the nervous system, organs, and cells.

According to William Philpott, M.D., a magnetic therapy pioneer of Choctaw, Oklahoma, when used properly, magnetic field therapy has no known harmful side effects. Dr. Philpott has found that the "negative magnetic field" can even reverse cancer. (A compass or magnetometer is used to identify the positive and negative magnetic poles").

"Whether it is a cut, bruise, broken bone, infection or cancer, it is the negative magnetic energy that heals," Dr. Philpott states. He also points out that the same magnetic energy is capable of countering the toxic effects of poisonous chemicals, addictive drugs, and other potentially harmful substances.

The therapy is based on the fact that the body is surrounded by a magnetic field and is composed of numerous smaller magnetic fields, which become disturbed in the course of illness. Clinical research indicates that magnetic therapy can restore the body's normal, healthy magnetic fields and thereby promote recovery from cancer, says Dr. Philpott.

Positive magnetic energy possesses no capacity for regeneration or cancer reversal. The body must maintain a negative magnetic field in order for healing to occur.

The key to how magnetic fields can stimulate healing, and help in reversing cancer, has to do with its effect on oxygen, says Dr. Philpott. Magnetic fields can stimulate metabolism and increase the amount of oxygen available to cells. It has been speculated by Dr. Philpott have that oxygen deficiency, coupled with acidity, are unique characteristics of all cancer cells, and are actually the two main causes of cancer.

The more alkaline pH produced by a negative magnetic field is necessary for healing as cancer cannot grow in an alkaline environment, Dr. Philpott explains.

This common denominator is called **acid-hypoxia**, and refers to a cellular condition of acidity and low oxygen status. According to Dr. Philpott, cancer only develops in acid-hypoxia cellular tissue.

Numerous precipitating factors, such as carcinogens, excess free radicals, and maladaptive reactions to foods, geopathic stress, aberrant electromagnetic energy, and 60-cycle per second electrical pulsing frequency, can produce acidhypoxia.

This is when normal cells can turn to cancerous cells. A normal cell is alkaline, because otherwise oxygen could not be there for the cell to make its energy. A key chemical called adenosine triphosphate (ATP) is made by cells as an energy source through the use of oxygen; it is central to the way in which energy is released and transported.

This process is called oxidative phosphorylation and involves the addition of phosphate to adenosine, thereby creating high-energy phosphate bonds. Normal, healthy human cells use oxygen to produce ATP as an energy source.

Oxidative phosphorylation depends on conditions of alkalinity and high levels of molecular oxygen to function properly, says Dr. Philpott.

Infectious microorganisms (bacteria, fungi, and some intestinal parasites) and cancer cells have a different way of producing energy; it is called fermentative phosphorylation.

Here, under conditions of acidity and low or no oxygen, ATP is made through the fermentation of glucose (blood sugar) instead of through the use of oxygen. "In fact, if there were a lot of oxygen present, it would not work. Oxygen and the alkaline pH would inhibit this fermentation process, which requires a condition of acidity and no or low oxygen," explains Dr. Philpott.

Healthy human cells have the ability to make ATP by either method just described. However, fermentative phosphorylation cannot sustain life for humans but it will sustain the life of cancer cells, bacteria, fungi, and certain parasites. "The human bio-oxidative energy system is able to defeat the biological life energy system of cancer cells," he says.

Further, we get an estimated 10,000 injuries to our genetic material, or DNA, every day from carcinogenic chemicals. DNA can be repaired as long as the cells have plenty of oxygen and are alkaline; but if it is in an acid state it doesn't repair, and cancer cells can rapidly reproduce.

One other link involves a crucial series of enzymes. These enzymes help revert oxygen back to its normal molecular state where it can actively initiate normal oxidative phosphorylation process.

A positive magnetic field blocks the catalytic function of these enzymes and without sufficient negative magnetic energy acting as a kind of energy nutrient, the enzymes can't function to reverse conditions leading to cancer. "Thus, in addition to acid-hypoxia (oxygen shortage in acid conditions), a lack of negative magnetic energy can also be considered a major cause of cancer," Dr. Philpott states.

To defeat cancer, the cellular conditions must be changed so cancer cannot exist. Thus, the alkalinity and oxygen level in the cells must be raised with a negative magnetic field. A negative magnetic field applied to the human body has an amazing ability to remove cancerous conditions and replace them with an oxygen rich environment where cancer cells can't survive.

Magnetic field therapy can reduce the side effects of chemotherapy, and as previously mentioned positively influences the activity of enzymes. The negative magnetic field energy activates the oxidoreductase system, which is a highly efficient enzyme system that aids in detoxification. According to Dr. Philpott, "These systems turn harmful toxic acids into harmless and biologically necessary alkali substances. This then provides body cells with an abundance of necessary molecular oxygen for biological energy production."

**Clinical Guidelines for Treating Cancers with Magnetic Therapy:-**
The guidelines for treatment with this therapy require a physician's diagnosis and monitoring under the supervision of a Scientific Institutional Review Board.

**Magnetic Therapy** has been approved by the FDA and based on toxicity studies are classified as "not essentially harmful." Magnetic therapy for cancer continues to be considered experimental and warrants more studies. The indication is however, that a negative magnetic field has been observed in both animals and humans to reverse cancer lesions.

There is a bright future for patients who make choices for bettering their health and gaining complete healing through natural and alternative therapies. It is our greatest hope that you will have the confidence using this review as a guideline that these alternatives are the way to heal your body.

Here is a list from "An Alternative Medicine Definitive Guide to Cancer" by W. John Diamond, M.D. of Alternative cancer physicians. Much of the information from this publication has been used in this book.

Robert C. Adkins, M.D.          Keith Block, M.D.

The Atkins Center, 152 East 55th St.
New York, NY 10022
tel: 212-758-2110

W. John Diamond, M.D.
Triad Medical Center
4600 Kietzke Lane
M-242, Reno, NV 89502
tel: 702-829-2277

Steven B. Edelson, M.D.
3833 Roswell Rd, Ste. 110
Atlanta, GA 30342
tel: 404-841-0088

Tori Hudson, N.D.
A Woman's Time Natural Medicine
2067 N.W. Lovejoy
Portland, OR 97209
tel: 503-222-0276

Victor A. Marcial-Vega, M.D.
4037 Poinciana Ave.
Coconut Grove, FL 33133
tel: 305-442-1233

Emanuel Revici, M.D., Ken Korins M.D.
The Revici Life Science Center, Inc.
200 W. 57th St. Ste. 402
New York, NY 10019
tel: 212-246-5122

Geronimo Rubio, M.D.
American Metabolic Institute

Block Medical Center
1800 Sherman Ave.
Ste. 515, Evanston, IL 60201
tel: 847-492-3040

Douglas Brodie, M.D.
309 Kirman Ave, #2
Reno, NV 89502
tel: 702-324-7071

Patrick Donovan, M.D.
University Health Clinic
5312 Roosevelt Way NE
Seattle, WA 98105
tel: 206-525-8015

James W. Forsythe, M.D., H.M.D.
Cancer Screening and Treatment Center
75 Pringle Way, Ste. 909
Reno, NV 89502
tel: 702-329-5000

Dan Labriola, N.D.
P.O. Box 99157
Seattle, WA 98199
tel: 206-285-4993

Martin Milner, M.D.
Center For Natural Medicine, Inc.
1330 SE 39th Ave.
Portland, OR 97214
tel: 503-232-1100

Robert C. Rountree, M.D.
Helios Health Center

555 Saturn Blvd. Bldg B M/S 432
San Diego, CA 92154
tel: 619-267-1107

Charles B. Simone, M.MS., M.D.
Simone Protective Cancer Ctr
123 Franklin Corner Rd.
Lawrenceville, NJ 08648
tel: 609-896-2646

Jesse Stoff, M.D.
Solstice Clinical Associates
2122 N. Craycroft Road, #112
Tucson, AZ 85712
tel: 520-290-4516

Lawrence H. Taylor, M.D.
Advanced Medicine Center
1000 Cordova Court
Chula Vista, CA 91910
tel: 888-422-7434

International Listings

Ernesto R. Contreras, M.D.
Oasis Hospital, Tijuana No. 19
Apartado Postal No. 179
Playas de Tijuana, B.C. 22700
Mexico
tel: 5266-80-18 U.S 800-700-1850

Abram Hoffer, M.D. Ph.D.
2727 Quadra, Ste. 3
Victoria, British Columbia
Canada, V8T 4E5
tel: 250-386-8156

4150 Darley Ave. Ste. 1
Boulder, CO 80303
tel: 303-499-9224

Michael B. Schachter, M.D.
Schachter Ctr For Complementary Medicine
Two Executive Blvd., Ste. 202
Suffern, NY 10901
tel: 914-368-4700

Vincent Speckhart, M.D., M.D.H.
902 Graydon Ave, No 2
Norfolk, VA 23507
tel: 804-622-0014

Jack O. Taylor, M.S., D.C.
Dr. Taylor's Wellness Center, Inc.
3601 Algonquin Rd., Ste. 801
Rolling Meadows, IL 60008
tel: 847-222-1192

Etienne Callebout, M.D.
10 Harley Street
London, England W1N1AA
tel: 44-171-467-8300

**Physician Reference List:-** Following is a list of alternative and complementary practitioners (CAM) and doctors of good reputation, from around the world.

## Arizona

James Hutton, NMD. phone: (928) 203-9013; fax: (928) 203-9016
3510 Red Cliffs Lane, Sedona, AZ 86336

Sheldon C. Deal D.C., N.M.D., D.I.B.A.K. phone: (520) 323-7133; fax: (520) 323-8252  Chiropractic Kinesiologist
The Swan Clinic, 1001 North Swan Road, Tucson, Arizona 85711

Thomas Lodi, MD, MD(H). phone: (480) 834-5414; fax: (480) 834-5418; urgent: (480) 907-4419  Homeopath
An Oasis of Healing, Comprehensive Cancer Care, 210 North Center Street #102, Mesa, AZ 85201

Jesse Stoff, M.D. Solstice Clinical Associates, phone: (520) 290-4516; fax: (520) 290-6403
Southwest Professional Plaza, 2122 North Craycroft Road, #112, Tuscon, AZ 85712

Dr. Cyrus Wood-Thomas, D.N.B.H.E. phone: (866) 721-6091 Homeopath
10711 Oxbow Dr., Dewey AZ 86327

## Australia
Dr. Earl Owen, phone: (011) 61-2-9954-5455;  fax: (011) 61-02-9954-5055
Level 3, 121 Walker Street, North Sydney NSW 2060

## California

Madhuri Cawley, P.A-C., M.A., phone: (760) 295-5392; fax: (760) 295-5396
Health for Life, 2302 Amstel Lane, Vista, CA 92084

Dr. Mitchell R. Corwin (510) 845-3246  Chiropractic Kinesiologist
2914 Domingo Ave. Berkeley, CA 94705

James Dahlgren, MD, phone: (310).264.0234, fax: (310).449.5526 -- Internist and Toxicologist
BWell Clinic, 2811 Wilshire Blvd, #540, Santa Monica, CA 90403

Olaf Dietze, Director, HHP, CMT, OBT (707) 829-3537 Qigong
899 So. Gravenstein Hwy. Sebastopol, CA 95472

Gail M. Dubinsky, M.D. (707) 829-7596
1205 Gravenstein Hwy. S. Sebastopol, CA 95472

Patricia Ebert, D.C.  (818) 558-5613
2601 W Alameda Ave Ste 106 , Burbank , CA 91505

Elson M. Haas, M.D. (415) 472-2343
25 Mitchell Blvd. #8 San Rafael, CA 94903

Chris Henderson, ND, L.Ac. (707) 575-7505 Naturopathic and Acupuncture Optimal Health Center - 2464 W. Third St. Santa Rosa, CA 95401

Dr. Stephen Knight, ND, phone: (310) 988-8403, fax: (310).634-0389
Natural Health Partners, Inc, Torrance Medical Plaza, 3655 Lomita Blvd., Suite 308, Torrance, CA 90505

Dr. Michael Hollis, ND, phone: (310).264.0234, fax: (310).449.5526 -- Anti-Aging and Detoxification

BWell Clinic, 2811 Wilshire Blvd, #540, Santa Monica, CA 90403

Ron Kennedy, M.D. (707) 576-0100
2456 W. Third St. Santa Rosa, CA 95401

Dr. Cathie-Ann Lippman, M.D  (310) 289.8430 Autism, Cognitive Problems, Parkinson's, Epilepsy, Fibromyalgia, MS. The Lippman Center for Optimal Health, 291 S. La Cienega Blvd, Ste. 207, Beverly Hills, CA 90211

Sai-ling Michael, D.C. (818) 380-6830. 4560 Sherman Oaks Ave, Sherman Oaks, CA 91403

John Minye, D.D.S. (707) 539-8762. 4372 Sonoma Hwy. Santa Rosa, CA 95409

Carolyn Robertson, M.S., CEAP and Dr. Len Ochs, Ph.D. (510) 906-0420 Trauma 106 La Casa Via Suite 110, Walnut Creek, CA 94598

Geronimo Rubio, M.D. (619) 267-1107; fax: (619) 229-3003. American Metabolic Institute, 555 Saturn Blvd., Bldg B, M/S 432 San Diego, CA 92154

Simon Shapiro, L.Ac, phone: (310).264.0234, fax: (310).449.5526 -- Pain and Chinese Medicine. BWell Clinic, 2811 Wilshire Blvd, #540, Santa Monica, CA 90403

Aleksander Strande, ND., Ph.D. (949) 587-1513; Fax: (949) 587-1519 Simply Healing Clinic, 15520 Rockfield Blvd., Suite E1, Irvine, CA  92618

Lawrence Taylor, M.D. phone: (888) 626-8067. BioMedics Institute, 1000 Cordova Court, Chula Vista, CA 91910

Dr. Julian Whitaker, M.D. phone: US & Canada (800) 488-1500; all others: 949-851-1550. Whitaker Wellness Institute Medical Clinic, 4321 Birch St., Newport Beach, CA 92660

Matthew B. Zwerling, MD (707) 525-1311 Orthopedic and Surgery 4725A Hoen Ave., Santa Rosa, CA 95405

## Canada
Abram Hoffer, M.D. phone: (250) 386-8756; fax: (250) 386-5828 2727 Quadra, Suite 3, Victoria, British Columbia, Canada V8T 4E5

Anca Martalog, N.D. phone: (905) 884-7965; fax: (905) 884-0307 282 Elgin Mills Road W, Richmond Hill, Ontario, Canada

Patrick H. Ranch, D.C., M.D., N.M.D. (208) 777-8297 Photoluminescense or Ultraviolet Blood Irradiation (UBI). Clinic in British Columbia & Alberta

## Connecticut
Jeri Reid, phone 860.463.5109. Biological Blood Microscopy Education Inner Light Health & Wellness, Watkins Professional Center, 935 Main St. #4B Courtyard Rear, Manchester, CT 06040

## Colorado
Robert C. Rountree, M.D. phone: (303) 499-9224; fax: (303) 499-9593 Helios Health Center, 4150 Darley Avenue, Suite 1, Boulder, CO 80303

## Delaware
Robert Abel, Jr. M.D. phone: (302) 479-3937. Delaware Ophthalmology Consultants, Concord Plaza, 3501 Silverside Road, Wilmington DE 19810

Patricia Blanchfield CH, phone: (302) 588-0064. Hypnosis + Reiki Minds Eye Hypnosis, 5714 Kennett Pike, Unit R, Centreville, DE 19807

Laurie Dohmen VMD, phone 302-653-9970, fax (302) 659-5988. Holistic Veterinarian specializing in Acupuncture, nutrition, western herbs and Bach flower essences. Companion Animal Practice, 5121 DuPont Pkwy, Smyrna DE 19977

Shelley Epstein VMD, phone (302) 762-2694    Homeopathy + Raw Diet Wilmington Animal Hosp, 828 Phila Pike, Wilm 19809

Donald F. Feeney, D.C. phone: (302) 478-3028. Brandywine Total Health Care, 3214 Naamans Road, Wilmington, DE 19810

Albert Forwood, D.C., D.A.C.A.N. phone: (302) 778-0100. Concord Medical Chiropractic Neurology, 6 Sharpley Road at Route 202, Wilmington, DE 19803

Kathleen Gareth RN, MSN, FNP, phone: 302-478-7602 x3. Center for Integrative Health, 2502 Silverside Road #9, Wilmington, DE 19810

Dr. Julia Golod & Dr. Deana Burd, phone: 302-731-0869, 302-292-1777 Spinal Specialists of Delaware, 300 Christiana Medical Center, Christiana, DE 19702. Spinal Specialists of Delaware, 250 East Chestnut Hill Rd Newark, DE 19713

Polly Grimaldi, R.N. phone: (302) 454-1970. The Right Way by Polly, 416 New London Road, Newark, DE 19711

David Stanley Jezyk, M.D. phone: (302) 999.8901. 2055 Limestone Road #117, Wilmington, DE 19808

Aron Kerner, M.D. phone: (302) 428-1388; fax (303) 428-1379. 512 Greenhill Avenue, Wilmington, DE 19805

Jeff Kerner, M.D. phone: (302) 428-1388. 512 Greenhill Avenue, Wilmington, DE 19808

Chad Laurence D.C., phone (302) 234-1115; fax (302) 234-6661 Corrective Chiropractic, 7503-A Lancaster Pike, Hockessin, DE 19707

Lorna Lee, M. Ac, phone: 761-9095. The Massage Center, Philadelphia Pike, Wilmington, DE

Emil A. Mikhail, M.D. phone: (302) 778-0100. Concord Medical, 6 Sharpley Road at Route 202, Wilmington, DE 19803

P. Trent Ryan, D.C., D.A.C.N.B. phone: (302) 778-0100. Concord Medical Chiropractic Neurology, 6 Sharpley Road at Route 202, Wilmington, DE 19803

Gregory Serge, D.C. phone: (302) 239-8550. Hockessin Chiropractic, 424 Yorklyn Road, Suite 150, Hockessin, DE 19707

Alan Tillotson, PH.D; AHG; MA. phone: (302) 994-0565. Chrysalis Natural Medicine Clinic, 1008 Milltown Road, Wilmington, DE 19808

Seth Torregiani D.O. phone: (302) 266-9010. Omega Professional Center, J-30 Omega Drive, Newark, DE 19713

**England**
Etienne Callebout, M.D. phone: 44 (171) 467-8300; fax: 44 (171) 467-8312. 10 Harley Street, London, England V1N1AA or: 44 1582-769832

**Florida**
Scott Denny, DC, PhD, AP, FAAIM, phone (954) 473-8925; fax (954) 473-5993. MultiCare Rehabilitation, 2215 S. University Dr., Davie FL 33324

Victor A. Marcial-Vega, M.D. phone: (787) 598-0384. 4037 Poinciana Avenue, Coconut Grove, FL 33133

## Georgia
Stephen B. Edelson, M.D. phone: (404) 841-0088; fax: (404) 841-6416
3833 Roswell Road, Suite 110, Atlanta, GA 30342

## Illinois
Keith I. Block, M.D. phone: (847) 492-3040; fax: (847) 492-3045
Block Medical Center, 1800 Sherman avenue, Suite 515, Evanston, IL
60201

Dr. Dale Dunn, phone (708) 386-8822; fax (708) 848-1861
Synergy Health Systems, 6429 West North Avenue #101, Oak Park IL
60302

Dr. Vincent Hope, phone (815) 765-3727    Chiropractor, NRT (Nutritional
Response Therapy)
Poplar Grove, IL

## Massachusetts
James Belanger, M.D. phone: (781) 274-6190 -- prostate cancer survivor
since 1990 Focuses on immune system of cancer patients and unique
treatment plans designed to minimize effects of chemotherapy and
radiation Lexington Natural Health Center, 442 Marrett Rd, Suite 8,
Lexington, MA  02421

## Mexico
Geronimo Rubio, M.D. phone: (619) 267-1107; (800) 388-1083   [Psycho-
neuroimmunology and immunotherapy]. Saint Joseph Hospital, La Mesa,
Mexico -- **specializes in terminal cancer patients** --Can be reached
through the American Metabolic Institute 4364 Bonita Road #457, Bonita,
California 91902-1421

Ernesto R. Contreras, M.D. phone: 011-526-680-1850, (800) 700-1850; fax: (619) 297-3242. Chief Director and Founder of the Oasis Hospital, Paseo Playas #19, Tijuana, Mexico. Also PO Box 439045, San Ysidro, California 92143, U.S. phone: (800) 262-0212 (CA), (800) 523-8795 (US)

## New Hampshire
James D'Adamo, N.D. 44-46 Bridge Street, Portsmouth, NH 03801

## New Jersey
Michael Borokhovsky, pranic healer, phone:  (856) 216-7531
Pranic Healing & Meditation Center, 109 Spring Road, Cherry Hill, NJ 08003

Philip Getson, D.O. phone: (856) 596-5834, fax (609) 268-5763
Thermographic Diagnostic Imaging, 100 Brick Road, Suite 206, Southampton, NJ 08053

Charles B. Simone, M.D. phone: (609) 896-2646. Simone Protective Cancer Center, 123 Franklin Corner Rd., Lawrenceville, NJ 08648

Steven Streit, M.D. phone: (732) 367-5330; fax (732) 367-4394. 4710 Highway 9 S, Howell, NJ 07731

## New York
Emanuel Revici, M.D. phone: (212) 246-5122; fax: (212) 246-5711
The Revici Life Science Center, Inc., 200 West 57th Street #402, New York, NY 10019

Michael B. Schachter, M.D. phone: (845) 368-4700; fax: (845) 368-4727
Schachter Center for Complementary Medicine, 2 Executive Blvd #202, Suffern, NY 10901

## Nevada
W. John Diamond, M.D. phone: (702) 829-2277; fax: (702) 829-2365

Triad Medical Center, 4600 Kietzke Lane M242, Reno, NV 98502

James W. Forsythe, M.D. phone: (702) 826-9500; fax: (702) 329-6219
Century Wellness Center, 380 Brinkby Avenue, Reno, NV 89509

## Ohio

Theodore J. Cole, MA, DO, NMD phone: (513) 563-4321 x8325; fax (513)
777-1295  [Hyperbaric Oxygen]. The Cole Center for Healing, Inc, 11974
Lebanon Road, Suite 228, Cincinnati, OH 45241

Dr. Susan Jacobs, ND phone: (513) 563-4321; fax (513) 563-3131. The
Cole Center for Healing, Inc, 11974 Lebanon Road, Suite 228, Cincinnati,
OH 45241

WM. Westendorf, D.D.S. phone: (513) 923 3839; Fax: (513) 923 3853
Biological Dentistry. 2818 Blue Rock Road, Cincinnati, OH 45239

## Oregon

Dr. Brian Druker phone: (503) 494-9000; fax (503) 494-3688  CML
Oregon Health Sciences University, 3181 Sam Jackson Park Road,
Portland, OR 97201

Tkori Hudson, N.D. phone: (503) 222-2322; fax: (503) 222-0276
2067 N.W. Lovejoy, Portland, OR 97209

Martin Milner, N.D. phone: (503) 232-1100; fax: (503) 232-7751
Center for Natural Medicine, Inc., 1330 SE 39th Avenue, Portland OR
97214

## Pennsylvania

Anthony Bazzan, M.D, integrative physician, phone 610-630-8600; fax
610-630-9599. 2505 Blvd of the Generals, Jeffersonville, PA 19403

Ben Briggs, nutritionist, compounding pharmacist, phone: 610-363-7474; fax: 610-363- 5707. Lionville Natural Pharmacy, 309 Gordon Drive, Exton, PA 19341

Joel S. Edman, MS, D.Sc, nutritionist, phone 215-879-5121, fax: (215) 878-8358. Jefferson - Myrna Brind Center for Integrative Medicine, 925 Chestnut St, #120, Philadelphia, Pa 19107

Charlie Goedken, energy practitioner phone 717-558-8123. 506 Manor Terrace, Harrisburg, PA 17111

Dr Thomas L. Mather, ND, CTN, Dip.H.Ir, phone 570-934-0994; 607-725-4372. Mather Health Education Services, RR5 Box 5402, Montrose, PA 18801

Dr. Bernardo Merizalde, MD, phone 610-238-9963. (Mind, Body, Spirit) 600 Germantown Pike, Lafayette Hill, PA 19444

Dr. Kem Moser, biological dentist, phone 800-929-2844. 207 Market Street, Halifax, PA 17032

Frank C. Noonan, D.O. phone: (717) 733-1736. Central PA Integrative Medicine, 1248 West Main Street, Ephrata, PA 17522

Donald Robbins DMD, FAGD, AIAOMT phone (610) 3631980; fax (610) 363-7798. Dental Learning Resource, 340 North Route 100 POBox 449, Exton, PA 19341

Russell V. Silverman, D.O. phone (610) 388-3555; fax: (610) 388-3556 716 Woodward Road, Chadds Ford, PA 19317

Lynn Wright, RN, MSN, CM, MH, phone (570) 226-4222, fax (570) 226-2010 Live / Dry Microscopy, Bioterrain Auditing. Northern Light Healing Zone, 2591 Route 6 - Suite 104, Hawley, PA 18428

## Switzerland

Dr. Thomas Rau ++41 71 335 71 71, Fax ++41 71 335 7100
Paracelsus Klinik Lustmühle, 9062 Lustmühle (bei St. Gallen), Schweiz
CH-9062 Lustmühle near St.Gallen

Dr. Byron Braid ++41 71 335 71 71, Fax ++41 71 335 71 00
Paracelsus Klinik Lustmühle, 9062 Lustmühle (bei St. Gallen), Schweiz
CH-9062 Lustmühle near St.Gallen

## Tennessee

Damon Davidson, L.Ac.  phone: (423) 877-5001  Acupuncture, Chinese
Herbal Medicine, Medical Qigong Center for Traditional Medicine, 2145
Hamill Road, Chattanooga TN 37343

## Texas

Maxwell L. Axler, MD, FAAFP  phone: (713) 335-5697; fax: (713) 335-
5699 Burzynski Clinic, 9432 Old Katy Rd. Suite 200, Houston, TX 77055

Stanislaw R. Burzynski, M.D. phone: (713) 335-5697; fax: (713) 335-5699.
Cancer Burzynski Clinic, 9432 Old Katy Rd. Suite 200, Houston, TX 77055

Robert I. Lewy, MD, FACP  phone: (713) 335-5697; fax: (713) 335-5699.
Oncology Burzynski Clinic, 9432 Old Katy Rd. Suite 200, Houston, TX
77055

Robert A. Weaver, M.D.  phone: (713) 335-5697; fax: (713) 335-5699.
Internal Medicine Burzynski Clinic, 9432 Old Katy Rd. Suite 200, Houston,
TX 77055

## Virginia

Joan M. Resk, D.O.  phone (540) 776-8331. 5303 Clearbrook Village Lane,
Roanoke, VA 24014

Vincent Speckhart, M.D.  phone: (804) 622-0014; fax: (804) 622-9808
902 Graydon Avenue #2, Norfolk, VA 23507

## Washington
Patrick Donovan, N.D. phone: (206) 525-8015; fax: (206) 525-8014
University Health Clinic, 5312 Roosevelt Way NE, Seattle, WA 98105

George Gillson, MD  (253) 854-4900   Procarin Treatment for MS
Tahoma Clinic, 515 West Harrison, Kent, WA 98032

Dr. Gary Holz, D.Sc. (866) 474-9667  Psycho-neuroimmunology
Holz Health Center, Inc., 13588 Clayton Lane, Anacortes, WA. 98221

Dietrich Klinghardt, MD, Ph.D. phone: (425) 462-1777; fax: 425-453-
7015   Neural Therapy American Academy of Neural Therapy, PO Box
5023, Bellevue, WA 98004

Dan Labriola, N.D. phone: (206) 784-9111; fax: (206) 784-7444
Northwest Natural Health Specialty Care Clinic, 5343 Tallman Ave. NW,
Seattle, WA 98107

Charlotte Stuart, LAc  phone (206) 417-4785  Craniosacral Acupuncture --
Head & Back Trauma Specialist. Corelink Head and Back Center, 10522
Lake City Way, Suite C101, Seattle, WA 98125

Jonathan V. Wright, MD  (253) 854-4900 x 0. Tahoma Clinic, 515 West
Harrison, Kent, WA 98032

## Wisconsin
Geoffrey T. Bouc, MD (608) 365-7200. Bouc Family Wellness Center ,
3005 Riverside Beloit #101, Beloit, Wisconsin  53511

Following is a list of doctors who offer Ultraviolet Blood Irradiation (UBI) therapy.

## ALASKA
Sandra C. Denton, M.D. (907) 563-6200; fax: (907) 561-4933
Alaska Alternative Medicine Center, 3201 C Street #602, Anchorage, AK 99503

Robert Jay Rowen, M.D. (907) 344-7775; fax: (907) 522-3114. 615 E. 82nd Street, Suite 300, Anchorage, AK 99518

## ARIZONA
James Hutton, NMD. (928) 203-9013; fax: (928) 203-9016
3510 Red Cliffs Lane, Sedona, AZ 86336  jhutton@npgcable.com

Gordon Josephs, M.D. (602) 998-9232; fax: (602) 998-1528
7315 E. Evans Road, Scottsdale, AZ 85260

## CALIFORNIA
Randy S. Baker, MD  (831) 476-1886; fax: (831) 476-6198
1001 Hidden Valley Road, Soquel, CA 95073

Craig Jace ND, DOM, PA-C
10843 Magnolia Blvd, North Hollywood, CA 91601 (818) 505-8610

Dr. Jacob Swilling (619) 424-9552; fax: (619) 424-7593
Genesis West, 1161 Bay Blvd., Suite A, Chula Vista, CA 91911

## CANADA
Gordon E. Potter, MD (604) 534-5804; fax: (604) 534-7758
21693 52nd Avenue, Langley, B.C. V2Y1L7

Dr Tawnya Ward, Dr Eric Chan (604) 275 0163

Pangaea Clinic of Naturopathic Medicine, 120-12011 Second Ave, Richmond BC, Canada V7E 3L6

## CONNECTICUT
Dr. Robert M. Murphy (860) 482-4730; fax: (860) 482-9034
118 Migeon Avenue, Torrington, CT 06790

## FLORIDA
Martin Dayton, D.O. (305) 931-8484; fax: (305) 936-1849
18600 Collins Avenue, North Miami Beach, FL 33160

William Campbell Douglass,III, M.D., M.S. (888) 324-0888; fax: (407) 342-8222 The Douglass Center, 101 Timberlachen Circle #101, Lake Mary, FL 32746

Gary L. Pynckel, D.O. (941) 278-3377; fax: (941) 278-3702
3840 Colonial Blvd, Suite 1, Fort Myers, FL 33912

William N. Watson, M.D., PA (809) 623-3836
5536 Stewart St., Milton, FL 32570

## GEORGIA
Stephen B. Edelson, M.D. (404)841-0088; fax: (404) 841-6416
Environmental & Preventive Health Center, 3833 Roswell Rd, Street 110, Atlanta, GA 30342-4433

## IDAHO
Patrick H. Ranch, D.C., M.D., N.M.D. (208) 777-8297
Naturopahtic Clinic, 810 N. Henry, #230, Post Falls, m 83858
Also clinics in British Columbia & Alberta, Canada

## ILLINOIS
Ross A. Hauser, M.D. (708)848-7789; fax: (708) 848-7763

Caring Medical & Rehabilitation Services, 715 Lake Street, Suite 600, Oak Park, IL 60301

Jonathan Martinez D.O. (800) 981-9552; fax: (847) 255-7700
Pioneer Medical Associates, 3401 N. Kennicott Ave, Arlington Heights, IL 60004

## INDIANA
Dale Guyer, MD (317) 580-9355
Advanced Medical Center, 836 E 86th Street, Indianapolis, IN 46240

## JAPAN
Koichi Inoue, M.D. 81-3-5770-7737; fax: 81-3-5411-7479
Sanikoto-A1, 3-20-3, Kitame, Setagaya-Ku, Tokyo

## KANSAS
Jerry E. Block, M.D., F.A.C.P. (316) 251-2400; fax: (316) 251-1619
1501 W. 4th Street, Coffeyville, KS 67337

## MAINE
Arthur B. Weisser, D.O. (207) 873-7721; fax: (207) 873-7724
184 Silver Street, Waterville, ME 04901

## MARYLAND
Clinical Technology Center, 14816 Physicians Lane, Suite 151, Rockville, MD 20850. (301) 294-2928; fax: (301) 294-3195

Carl Schleicher, Ph.D. (301) 587-8686; fax: (301) 587-8688.
Foundation for Blood Irradiation, 1315 Apple Avenue, Silver Springs, MD 20910

## MEXICO
Dr. Amezcua 011-5266-301313; fax: 011-5266-301723
Genesis West, 256 Del Agua, Tijuana, BC 22880

Dr. Cesar Garcia, Chief of Staff 011-5266-801358; fax: 011-52-66-801831
Hospital Meridien, Lava #2971 Secc. Costa Hermosa, Playas de Tijuana,
BC, CP22240 Mexico

Frank J. Morales Jr., M.D. 011-5288-124842
Ave. Alvaro Obregon # 77, Col.Jardin C.P. 87330, H. Matamoros, Tamps.
MEX

Frank J. Morales Jr., M.D. (99) 23-33-33
Morales Clinic, Calle 57 No.500 entre 58y60, Merida, Yuc. MEX
Mailing Address: 1424 W. Price Rd., Suite 450, Brownsville, TX 78520

Coahuila Con Benito Juarez 011-5298-370159
No.6 "A", Nuevo Progreso, Tamps. MEX

**MICHIGAN**
Vahagn Agbabian, D.O. (248) 334-2424; fax: (248) 334-2924
N.B.A. Building, 28 Saginaw, Street 1105, Pontiac, MI 48304

John O. Wycoff, D.O. (517) 333-7270 (800) 471-0255
1226 Michigan Avenue, East Lansing, MI 48823

**NEVADA**
David A. Edwards, MD, HMD (775) 828-4055; fax: (775) 828-4255
6490 South McCarran Blvd, Suite 24, Reno, NV, 89509

Robert D. Milne, M.D. (702) 385-1393; fax: (702) 385-4170
Milne Medical Center, 2110 Pinto Lane, Las Vegas, NV 89106

**NEW HAMPSHIRE**
Dr. Irma Barkan fax: (603) 472-5962
15 Constitution Drive, Bedford, NH 03110, (603)472-5007

## NEW JERSEY
Ivan Krohn, M.D. (866) 987-5433; fax: (732) 506-6039
Longevity Medical, 540 Bordentown Avenue, Suite 4200, South Amboy, NJ

Stuart L. Weg, M.D. (201) 447-5558; fax: (201) 447-9011
Pain Relief & Treatment Specialists, 1250 E. Ridgewood Ave, Ridgewood, NJ 07450

## NEW YORK
Steven Bock, M.D. + Kenneth Bock, M.D. (914) 876-7082; fax: (914) 876-4615 Rhinebeck Health Center, 108 Montgomery Street, Rhinebeck, NY 12572

Center For Progressive Medicine, Pinnancle Place, Suite 210, 10 McKown Road, Albany, NY 12203.
(518) 435-0082; fax: (518) 435-0086

Mitchell Kurk, M.D. (516) 239-5540; fax: (516) 371-2919
310 Broadway, Lawrence, NY 11559

Thomas K Szulc, M.D. (516) 931-1133; fax: (516) 931-1167
Long Island Pain Treatment Center, 720 Old Country Road, Plainview, NY 11803

## NORTH CAROLINA
Dennis W. Fera, MD (919) 732-2287; fax: (919) 732-3176
Holistic Health & Medicine, 1000 Corporate Dr., Suite 209, Hillsborough (Chapel Hill), NC 27278

Bhaskar D. Power, M.D., FRCS (919) 535-1411; fax: (919) 537-5000
Genesis Health Center, 1201 East Littleton Road, Roanoke Rapids, NC 27870

## OHIO

Theodore J. Cole, M.A., D.O., N.M.D., F.A.A.I.M. (513) 563-4321; fax: (513) 563-3131.
The Cole Center for Healing, 11974 Lebanon Road, Cincinnati, OH 45241

## OKLAHOMA
Leon Anderson, D.O. (918) 299-5038; fax: (918) 299-5038
Anderson Clinic, P.O. Box 1032 - 121 S. Second St., Jenks, OK 74037

Charles H. Farr, M.D., Ph.D. (405) 634-7855; fax: (405) 634-7320
Genesis Medical Research Institute, 5419 5. Western Ave, Oklahoma City, OK 73109

Gordon P. Laird, D.O. (918) 762-3601; fax: (918) 762-2544
Alpha Health, 304 Boulder, Pawnee, OK 74058

Robert L. White, N.D., Ph.D., PA-C (405) 634-7855; fax: (405) 634-7320
Genesis Medical Research Institute, 5419 So. Western Ave, Oklahoma City, OK 73109

## PENNSYLVANIA
Andrew Lipton, DO (610) 667-4601; fax: (610) 667-6416
822 Montgomery Ave., Suite 315, Narberth, PA 19072

## TAIWAN
Kojak Lin, MD (886) 7-3485858; Fax: (886) 7-3486888
14 Min-Ren Road, Kaohsiung, Taiwan

## TEXAS
Dr. Barry Beaty. (817) 737-6464; fax: (817) 737-2858
4455 Camp Bowie Blvd, Suite 211, Fort Worth, TX 76107-3800

Charles M. Hawes, D/C + Antonio Acevdeo, D/C (817) 446-8416; fax: (817) 446-8413. Preventive Medicine Center, 6451 Brentwood Stair Rd, Suite 115, Ft. Worth, TX 76112

John. L. Sessions, D.O. (409) 423-2166; fax: (409) 423-5496.
1609 5. Margaret, Kirbyville, TX 75956

**WASHINGTON**
Cheryl M. Deroin, N.D.
3606 Main Street, Suite 202, Vancouver, WA 98663

---

If you would like to find a physician that uses a **combination of alternative and conventional** therapy to treat your cancer, the following physicians use both:

Keith Block, M.D. at the Block Medical Center in Evanston, IL uses a complete detoxification program along with both conventional and complementary techniques.

Dr. Brodie in Reno includes nutritional and herbal supplements along with strong physical and psychological support and conventional treatments where necessary.

**The Buchholz Medical Group** in Mt View treats cancer, primarily with chemo emphasizing the prevention of side effects, and control of symptoms form the illness and from treatment. Traditional Chinese medicine is available, including acupuncture and herbal medicine. They will combine alternative and conventional. Phone: (415) 988-8011.

**Energy Health Centre** Ft. Worth, Texas offers integrative treatments that combine conventional and complementary medicine in the healing of cancer. They have a website at http://www.energyhealth.com/ and can be reached by phone at 817-927-5111.

James W. Forsythe, M.D., H.M.D. manages two clinics: Cancer Screening and Treatment Center of Nevada for conventional cancer treatment and Century Wellness Center for alternative medicine. Dr. Forsythe's expertise is in conventional therapy and he may propose that as your first option.

Humlegaarden is an international cancer clinic situated north of Copenhagen in Denmark, using innovative and holistic methods in the treatment of cancer. In some cases, chemotherapy may be used.

Klinik St. George in Germany uses hyperthermia with a variety of conventional and alternative approaches.

Dan Labriola, N.D., in Seattle works with patients who need or want to stay with conventional treatments and uses naturopathic approaches to provide nutritional supplementation to help reduce the side effects of chemotherapy and other harsh treatments.

**North Central Mississippi Regional Cancer Center** in Greenwood, MS incorporates bromocryptine, coQ10, and other immune system boosting agents with traditional cancer therapy. They can be reached by phone at 601-459-7133.

**Northern Health Inc.** in Ontario - Rudolf E. Falk, M.D., may use low-dose chemotherapy, non-steroidal anti-inflammatory drugs, and high doses of vitamin C, all of which are combined with hyaluronic acid, which is a targeting carrier molecule.

The use of hyaluronic acid allows for better penetration of the drug to the tumor, and also better targeting, so the severe side effects of drugs are not felt. They may also use hyperthermia. Phone: (705)466-2015.

Oasis of Hope in Mexico uses mostly alternative therapies, but in some cases, such as with liver cancer, they may combine conventional therapies. With liver cancer, they combine 5FU (chemotherapy) with laetrile and inject it directly into the liver.

They are having some good success with this. In addition, they have a **4 Day Program for** people **doing chemotherapy** who want to complement it with alternative approaches

Revici Clinic uses non-toxic chemotherapy for treating late stage cancers.

**University Heights Cancer Center** Indianapolis, Indiana is a complete facility for cancer treatment. This facility may not be considered alternative, except for their use of hyperthermia, an advanced method that enhances the effect of cancer therapy with minimal side effects. They can be reached at (317) 297-2684 or by email at shidnia@earthlink.net.

Meridian Energy Therapies (METs) became a separate healing field when a US psychologist, Dr Roger Callahan, began to use insights about the body's energy system to treat psychological problems with astonishing success in the early 1980s.

A large part of METs is still devoted to treating psychological problems such as fear, phobias, anxieties, motivation problems etc. This is also known as "Energy Psychology" and this rapidly developing field is re-writing the definitions of what is causing mental disturbances and how to treat such disturbances swiftly, gently and very effectively.

Originally, there were only a few separate techniques. But in recent years, active research and feedback by a large number of innovators who came from other fields of human healing and found in the new Meridian Energy Therapies answers and routes of enquiry that were simply not available before has created a wonderful variety of METs.

The following Members have been certified by the **Association for Meridian Energy Therapies** (The AMT) as Meridian Energy Therapy Practitioners. This qualification also includes intensive knowledge of Emotional Freedom Techniques (EFT).

Sebnem Akalin. Istanbul, Turkey. Cell # 90 530 517 75 40

Ilknur Akarsu. Turkey. Phone +90 532 495 76 18

Fatime Akgöz. Izmir, Turkey. Phone +90 505 708 95 55

Cigdem Akin. Istanbul, Turkey. Phone 0533 308 23 82

Nazmiye Akyıldız. Istanbul, Turkey. Phone +90 505 400 94 36

Aynur Apaydin. İstanbul, Turkey. Phone 0 532 733 31 05

Karen Aquinas. Oregon, United States. www.biofieldhealthservices.com

Gulcan Arpacioglu Adams. Istanbul, Turkey. Phone 902163023865 or Cell # 532 503 1776

Cagatay Atasagun. Istanbul, Turkey. Phone 0533 337 4444

Murat Aydın. Kayseri, Turkey. Phone +90 533 657 3297

GÜl Aytekİn Özen. İstanbul, Turkey. Phone 90 533 248 30 15

Alan Balfour. West Yorkshire, England. Phone 0113 2585438

Mathilde Barbier. Surrey, England. Phone ( 44) 07947 319 362

Tina Beckham. Kent, England. Ashford, Kent, England

Wendy Leanne Beresford. Gloucestershire, England. Phone 07855699463

Jacqueline Besseling. Nederland. Prof. Evertslaan 130b. 2628 XZ Delft. 06

125 843 48 or E-mail: jacqueline.besseling@gmail.com

Wendy Birse. Perth and Kinross, Scotland. Cell # 07774 813 178

Arzu Bıyıklı. Ataşehir, Turkey. Phone +90 533 322 19 78

Joanne Blachut. Queensland, Australia.

https://joanneblachut.goe.ac/contact/

Shiloh Blachut. Queensland, Australia.

https://shilohblachut.goe.ac/contact/

Gisèle Bourgoin. Québec, Canada. Phone 418-651-5938

Susan Browne. Co. Kerry, Ireland. Phone 00353 863381850

Joyce Bunton. Glasgow, Scotland. Phone 07939 984 602.

Stephen Carter. Maryland, United States. Phone 1-804-677-6772

Maria Chappell. South Yorkshire, England. Phone 07971 463324

Vivian Choi. Cambridgeshire, England. https://vivianchoi.goe.ac/contact/

Toks Coker. London, England. Phone 07973210107

Ber Collins. County Clare, Ireland. Phone 00353868103342

Mikael Cormont. Paris, France. Cell # 33 (0)6 27 46 01 10

Natalie Cowell. East Sussex, England. Phone 01273562649 or Cell # 07811378087

Paula Cowell. West Sussex, England. Cell # 07919 201640

Ina Maria D'Costa. Swindon, England. Phone 01793 850499

Patricia Dancing-Elk-Walls. Texas, United States.

https://patriciadancingelk-walls.goe.ac/contact/

http://patriciawalls.net/

Grace DaSilva-Hill. Kent, England. Cell # 07590524795

Tanya Davies. Queensland, Australia. Phone 0420502722

Clare Davison. West Sussex, England. Phone 01403 734 930

Nanouschka de Wilde. Manchester, England. Phone 0161 799 6700 or Cell # 07708028278

Janet Deane. County Donegal, Ireland. https://janetdeane.goe.ac/contact/

Esen Dedeoglu. İzmir, Turkey. Phone +90 5334599781

Fiona Dilston. Edinburgh City, Scotland. Phone 07753505292

Peter Donn. Hertfordshire, England. Phone 01923 260 050

Hayley Driscoll. Cardiff, Wales. Phone 07949327385

Paula Duarte. London, England. Cell # 07845037563

Fatma El Sayed. Cairo, Egypt. Phone +20(0)1111 821271 or

Cell # 2(0)1111821271

Rania El Tahtawy. Cairo, Egypt. Cell # 201097098047

Mariam Emara. Cairo, Egypt. Phone +20 10 985 97003

Sabiha Erdinc. Marmaris, Turkey. Phone +90252 4171200 or

Cell # +905383660634

Gülüm Erdinç. Istanbul, Turkey. Phone +90 536 233 24 28

Berat Yeliz Eren. İstanbul, Turkey. Phone +90 533 272 57 12

Hayriye Erhan. Kayseri, Turkey. Phone +90 (0)541 243 4812

Tansu Erkan. Istanbul, Turkey. Phone 0535 358 81 65

Saliha Eroglu. Turkey, Turkey. Phone 90 532 423 15 72 or Cell #

905433304923

Naglaa Ezzat. Cairo, Egypt. Phone +20(0)1110505566

Lidia Ferreira. São Domingos De Rana, Cascais, Portugal.

https://lidiaferreira.goe.ac/contact/

Lorna Firth. Paphos, Cyprus. Phone +357 26934319 or

Cell # +357 99479426

Nelle Flynn. New South Wales, Australia. Phone +61 266777509

Davide Focardi. Co. Kildare, Ireland. Phone +353 87 6229714

Margarita Foley. Dublin, Ireland. Phone 00353863553981

Amanda Freeman. VIC, Australia. Phone 0438 668 688 or

Cell # 0438 668 688

Françoise Gins. Oxfordshire, England. Cell # 07958 131132

Philip Gowler. Berkshire, England. philgowler.co.uk.

https://philipgowler.goe.ac/contact/

Caner Gözütok. Adana, Turkey. Phone +90 532 356 58 08

Hülya Gürsözer Coşğun. Istanbul, Turkey. Phone 90 533 486 50 24

Funda Haberal. Istanbul, Turkey. Phone 05423417773

Silvia Hartmann. East Sussex, England. silviahartmann.com -

https://energyart.uk/

Saziye Hayat Etingu. Istanbul, Turkey. Phone 0216 350 01 21 or

Cell # 0533 551 51 45

Sandra Hillawi. Hampshire, England. Phone +44 (0)2392 433 928 or

Cell # 07884 443 708

Marion Hind. Northamptonshire, England. Cell # 07432 617491

Nicola Hok. London, England. Phone +44 (0)7415 88 99 63

Michaela Hope. Hampshire, England. Phone 07982 838460 or

Cell # 07982 838460

Sevil İlgün. Istanbul, Turkey. Phone +90 553 612 71 73

Kirsten Ivatts. Derbyshire, England. Phone 01335 390638 or

Cell # 07805 925275

Denise Jacques. County Durham, England.

https://denisejacques.goe.ac/contact/

Ferris Jay. County Leitrim, Ireland. Cell # 00 353 89 4171388

Katerina Kalchenko. Ukraine, Ukraine. https://happykaterina.com/ or

https://katerinakalchenko.goe.ac/contact/

Nesrin Kandemir. Istanbul, Turkey. Phone +90 532 220 44 62

Gülsun Kemaloğlu. Istanbul, Turkey. Phone +90 541 668 92 77 or

Cell # 90 541 6689277

Susan Kennard. East Sussex, England. Phone 07737100254 or

Cell # 01424715631

Aisling Killoran. Dublin, Ireland. Phone 01 2986507 or

Cell # 087 1352 122

Silvia King. East Sussex, England. https://silviaking.goe.ac/contact/

Aysun Kıran. Istanbul, Turkey. Phone +90 545 769 51 35 or

Cell # 05539457677

Dilek Kirikkanat. Turkey, Turkey. Phone 0507 245 9785 or

Cell # 00905302306226

Şebnem Koral. Bursa, Turkey. https://sebnemkoral.goe.ac/contact/

Irene Lambert. Derbyshire, England. Phone +44 (0)1332 863 290 or
Cell # 07903 711 079

Agnes Lau. Singapore, Singapore. http://www.mindtransformations.com/

or https://agneslau.goe.ac/contact/

Kym Lawn. Queensland, Australia. Phone 0406 182 735 or

Cell # 0406 182 735

Isaac Lim. Selangor, Malaysia. http://www.eftwonder.com/ or

https://isaaclim.goe.ac/contact/

Maria LiPuma. Oregon, United States. http://www.noble-being.com/

Irene Loudon. England. Phone 01413328829

Teresa Lynch. New Jersey, United States. Phone 908.431.0092

Katherine Lynch. New Jersey, United States. Phone 908-904-4657

Yvonne Maclean. Surrey, England. Phone 07814619265

Ray Manning. Dublin, Ireland. Phone 00353-1- 298 6507 or

Cell # 00353 87 677 8049

Denise Marchisotto. New Jersey, United States. Cell # 732.718.1818

Kelly Mayne. England. Phone 07879332394

Helen McCrarren. Monaghan, Ireland.

http://www.mindbodyenergymatters.ie/ or

https://helenmccrarren.goe.ac/contact/

Siadbh McGivern. West Cork, Ireland. Phone 00353 876104498

Bridin McKenna UKCP Reg. Clinical Psychotherapist. Belfast, Northern Ireland. Phone 07706705814 or

https://bridinmckenna.goe.ac/contact/

Michael Millett. Lincolnshire, England. Phone 01476 568800 or Cell # 0845 6588220

Laura Moberg. New Hampshire, United States. Cell # 1 (603) 359-4782

Sharon Moore. New Jersey, United States. Phone 609-937-0502

Patricia Moreby. Warwickshire, England. Cell # 07977 099027

Tracy Morrow. Berkshire, England. Phone 01635 44200 or Cell # 07967 340479

Auk Murat. Jawa Barat, Indonesia. Phone +6281802177777

Prabha Nagaraja. Delhi, India. https://twitter.com/@PrabNag

Karen Neil. County Durham, England. Cell # 0774 7831 850

Özlem Öğüç. Istanbul, Turkey. Phone +90 532 227 13 81

Cumasiye Ozgur. İzmir, Turkey. Phone +905303869748

Erkan Özkan. Istanbul, Turkey. Phone +90 554 958 16 44

Nimet Özkan. Istanbul, Turkey. Phone 90 554 958 16 47 or

Cell # 05549581647

Alexandra Paulino. Portugal, Portugal. Phone +351 96 610 7832 or

Cell # 96 610 78 32

António Rebocho. Lisboa, Portugal. Phone 351 933 375 724

Aleksandra Rechtman. London, England. Phone 07920746442

Eric Robins. California, United States. Phone 310 872 7446

Jonah Robins. California, United States. Phone 310 987 8874

Seda Rodop Soran. Istanbul, Turkey. Phone 0090 (212) 296 0008

Gizela Rodrigues. Lisboa, Portugal. Phone +351 965 806 862 or

Cell # 96 580 68 62

Lauren Rosenberg. London, England. Phone 07966268148

Helen Ryle. Co. Kerry, Ireland. Phone 00353 87 773 4914

Iman Saad. Cairo, Egypt. Cell # 01005838109

Sevgi Şahin. Istanbul, Turkey. Phone 90 0532 262 95 08 or

Cell # 0905322629508

Barbara Saph. Hampshire, England. Phone 02380 663 658 or

Cell # 07919 162 542

Heidi Saputelli. Beinwil am See, Switzerland. Phone 062 772 02 34 or

Cell # 079 578 81 08

Gamze Sari. Merkez Yalova, Turkey. Phone +905330282844

İpek Şekerdil. İzmir, Turkey. Phone +90 507 866 05 89

Sevim Sanem Selametoglu Ozcan. Antalya, Turkey.

Cell # 00905071767606

Keren Shamay. Texas, United States. Phone 1-682-233-1412

Sandra Smith. County Dublin, Ireland. Phone 00353 -86-3130969

Sadullah Sönmez. Kayseri, Turkey. Phone +90 535 270 7794 or

Cell # 905352707794

Eliezer Spetter. Jerusalem, Israel. Phone +972 29 943 704 or

Cell # 00 972 545 340 155

John Staples. Maryland, United States. Phone 703-283-5177

Dave Stewart. Greater Manchester, England. Phone 01616219653 or

Cell # 07766487194

Şengül Sürmen. Istanbul, Turkey. Phone 90 533 743 15 81

Evgenia Sverbikhina. FL, United States.

https://evgeniasverbikhina.goe.ac/contact/ or

https://evgeniasverbikhina.goe.ac/contact/

Emel Talay. İzmir, Turkey. Phone +90 532 367 04 58

Sam Thorpe. East Sussex, England. https://samcoxthorpe.goe.ac/contact/

or http://www.conscioushealthpractice.com/

Filiz Topaçlıoğlu. Ankara, Turkey. Phone +90 555 997 97 07

Sally Topham. Norfolk, England. Phone 020 7604 3619

Janine Turner. Kent, England. https://janineturner.goe.ac/contact/

Jamesylvester Urama. Nigeria. Phone 07405223058

Emmy Vadnais. Minnesota, United States. Phone 651-292-9938

Jorge Vence. Hampshire, England. Phone 07914016397 or

Cell # 07914016397

Nanette L Waller. Oklahoma, United States. Phone 918 682 6941

Ilka Wandel. Alicante, Spain. https://ilkawandel.goe.ac/contact/

Barney Wee. Singapore, Singapore. Phone +65 9667 8696

Deborah Wiggins-Hay. Herefordshire, England. Phone 07875751890 or

Cell # 07875751890

Donna Wirth. Pennsylvania, United States. Cell # 724-516-0583

Reto Wyss. Berne, Switzerland. Phone +41 62 962 9212

Aysenur Yabanigul. Istanbul, Turkey.

https://aysenuryabanigul.goe.ac/contact/

Eda Yaman. Adana, Turkey. Phone +90 543 717 22 87

Gülbahar Yeni. Turkey, Turkey. Phone +90(0) 232 336 6445 or

Cell # +90(0)532 665 5980

Beyza Yücel. Kayseri, Turkey. Phone +90 (0)532 428 0172

Ahmad Zabihi. Tehran, Iran. Phone +989121719046 or

Cell # 0757 0066556

Suzanne Zacharia. Kent, England. Phone 07533636939 or

Cell # 07533636939

Daniela Ziehn. Wesel, Germany. Phone 00492814607472 or

Cell # 00491787986773

**Poly MVA:-** is a new, nontoxic, powerful antioxidant formula that **protects** both cellular DNA and RNA.

The scientifically designed mechanism of action is to "fix the cell" and control the cancer, rather than "fight the cancer" and poison the system as noted above.

**Poly MVA** offers an extremely powerful alternative cancer treatment without the toxic side effects associated with most Conventional Cancer Treatments.

Doctors (See Practioners List below) and **Patients worldwide** are reporting the benefits of **Poly MVA** when used as a stand-alone option or when used in conjunction with Chemotherapy and Radiation.

**POLY MVA** has been scientifically designed to **CORRECT DNA BREAKDOWNS** and return the damaged cell to normal cellular function.

This product was developed by **Dr. Merrill Garnett**, a highly regarded biochemist, who has been conducting research with the objective of creating an electronic frequency specificity to restore the DNA exchange energy pathway.

**Poly-MVA**(LAPd) compounds transfer current inward from the cell membrane phospholipid to DNA via the mitochondria.

This high flux state of inward pulsed current maintains normal electron oxygen transport, but can be shown to electrically dissociate (breakdown) membranes of primitive anaerobic (CANCER) cells including amoeba, yeasts, and certain tumors.

**ALABAMA**

**Larry D. Brock, MD**

**Regenerative Medicine Center**
5901 Airport Blvd. Suite E. Mobile, Alabama 36608-3156
Ph:251-342-0505
Fax: 251-342-0360
email: drbrock@regenerativemedicine-al.com
Website: www.bioidenticalhormonemd.com

---

## ALASKA

**Gary Geraly, M.D.**
615 East 82nd Ave., Suite 300
Anchorage, Alaska, 99518
Phone: (907)-344-7775
Fax: (907)-522-3114
E-Mail: compmed@alaska.net

---

## ARIZONA

Robert Zieve, MD
EuroMed Foundation
34975 N. North Valley Parkway
Bldg. 6, Suite 138
Phoenix, Arizona 85086
Phone: 602-404-0400
Fax: 602-404-0403
Website: www.euro-med.us

Harvey Abrams, DC

Rehabilitation Chiropractic Care
801 S. Power Road #107
Mesa, AZ 85206
Phone: 480-396-4400
Fax: 480-218-9324
Website: http://rehabchiro.com
Email: drabrams@rehabchiro.com

Martha Grout, MD, MD(H)
Arizona Center for Advanced Medicine
9328 E. Raintree Drive
Scottsdale, AZ 85260
Phone: (480)-240-2600
E-Mail: drmartha@arizonaadvancedmedicine.com

Charles H. Baughman, MD
Baughman & Associates Age Management Medicine
1366 N. 94th Dr. Suite E1
Peoria, AZ 85381
Phone: 623-977-0955
Fax: 623-977-3729
E-mail: crsgsdoc@cox.net
Website: www.growyounger.us

Ronald Peters, MD
MindBody Medicine Center
13951 N. Scottsdale Road
Scottsdale, AZ 85254
Phone: (480) 607-7999

Dean Silver, MD
7420 Pinnacle Road Suite 126
Scottsdale, AZ 85255
Phone: (480) 860-0689

Website: www.deansilvermd.com

## CALIFORNIA

Antonio Jimenez, MD
Hope 4 Cancer Institute
13910 Lyons Valley Road, Suite L
Jamul, CA 91935
Phone: 855-366-4673
Fax: 619-956-7071
Website: www.h4cmedical.com
Email: info@h4cmedical.com

Ron Rothenberg, MD
California Healthspan Institute
320 Santa Fe Dr, #211, Encinitas, CA 92024
Phone: (760) 635-1996

Shivinder Deol, MD (Diplomate, Anti-Aging Medicine)
Anti-Aging & Wellness Center
4000 Stockdale Hwy., Suite D
Bakersfield, CA 93309
Phone: (661) 325-7452
Fax: (661) 325-7456
E-mail: doc@drdeol.com
Website: www.drdeol.com

Areas of specialty: Alternative and complementary medicine, IV vitamin C, hyberbaric oxygen, pH balance, Poly-MVA and more.

James L. Padilla, D.C.
San Diego Spine and Wellness Center
12070 Carmel Mtn. Rd. Ste. 290
San Diego, CA 92128

Phone: (858)676-1166
E-Mail: Linda@DrJamesPadilla.com
Website: http://www.DrJamesPadilla.com

Mezia O. Azinge-Obasi, MD
Doctor Paul Memorial Medical Center, Inc.
3450 W. 43rd Street, Suite 106
Los Angeles, CA. 90008
Phone: (323)290-2832
Fax: (323)290-2836
E-mail: dr.paul@dslextreme.com
Website: www.dromd.com
Areas of specialty: Care of the under-served, integrating Anti-Aging
Medicine and Alternative Medicine with Conventional Family Medicine to
achieve affordable balanced health. These include common Herbs,
Vitamins, Minerals, Hormones, pH balance, attention to blood type
differences, eating habits and more.

William S. Eidelman, MD
The Center For Healing & Transformation
(Programs for Healing Serious Illnesses)
1654 N. Cahuenga Blvd.
Los Angeles, CA 90028
Phone: 323-463-3295
Fax: 323-463-3740
E-mail: williameidelman@gmail.com
Websites: www.DrEidelman.com

Dr. Kristine Reese
LotusRain Naturopathic Clinic
5210 Balboa Ave Ste F
San Diego, CA 92117
Phone: 619-239-5433
Website: hwww.lotusrainclinic.com/

Gary Foresman, MD
Middle Path Medicine
180 W. LePoint Street Unit A
Arroyo Grande, CA 93420
Phone: (805) 481-3442
Website: www.middlepathmedicine.com

Brent Hill, DC
Hill Center for Integrated Medicine
3609 Oakdale Rd., Suite 5
Modesto, CA 95357
Phone: (209) 551-8888
Website: www.hillwellness.com/

Paul Han Soo Kim, MD
Previ Medical Group
1776 Ygnacio Valley Rd., Suite 204
Walnut Creek, CA 94598
Phone: 925-691-7546
Website: www.previmedicalgroup.com/index.html

Leigh Erin Connealy, MD
Cancer Center for Healing
6 Hughes, Suite 120B
Irvine, CA 92618
Phone: 949-581-HOPE (4673)
E-mail: info@cancercenterforhealing.com
Website: www.cancercenterforhealing.com

Area of specialty: Targeted cancer therapies including IPTLD, high-dose vitamin C, hyperbaric oxygen therapy, ultraviolet blood irradiation, light beam generator, nutraceuticals, surgery, emotional therapies and more.

**CALIFORNIA**

Antonio Jimenez, MD
Hope 4 Cancer Institute
13910 Lyons Valley Road, Suite L
Jamul, CA 91935
Phone: 855-366-4673
Fax: 619-956-7071
Website: www.h4cmedical.com
Email: info@h4cmedical.com

Ron Rothenberg, MD
California Healthspan Institute
320 Santa Fe Dr, #211, Encinitas, CA 92024
Phone: (760) 635-1996

Shivinder Deol, MD (Diplomate, Anti-Aging Medicine)
Anti-Aging & Wellness Center
4000 Stockdale Hwy., Suite D
Bakersfield, CA 93309
Phone: (661) 325-7452
Fax: (661) 325-7456
E-mail: doc@drdeol.com
Website: www.drdeol.com

Areas of specialty: Alternative and complementary medicine, IV vitamin C, hyberbaric oxygen, pH balance, Poly-MVA and more.

James L. Padilla, D.C.
San Diego Spine and Wellness Center
12070 Carmel Mtn. Rd. Ste. 290
San Diego, CA 92128
Phone: (858)676-1166
E-Mail: Linda@DrJamesPadilla.com

Website: http://www.DrJamesPadilla.com

Mezia O. Azinge-Obasi, MD
Doctor Paul Memorial Medical Center, Inc.
3450 W. 43rd Street, Suite 106
Los Angeles, CA. 90008
Phone: (323)290-2832
Fax: (323)290-2836
E-mail: dr.paul@dslextreme.com
Website: www.dromd.com

Areas of specialty: Care of the under-served, integrating Anti-Aging Medicine and Alternative Medicine with Conventional Family Medicine to achieve affordable balanced health. These include common Herbs, Vitamins, Minerals, Hormones, pH balance, attention to blood type differences, eating habits and more.

William S. Eidelman, MD
The Center For Healing & Transformation
(Programs for Healing Serious Illnesses)
1654 N. Cahuenga Blvd.
Los Angeles, CA 90028
Phone: 323-463-3295
Fax: 323-463-3740
E-mail: williameidelman@gmail.com
Websites: www.DrEidelman.com

Dr. Kristine Reese
LotusRain Naturopathic Clinic
5210 Balboa Ave Ste F
San Diego, CA 92117
Phone: 619-239-5433
Website: hwww.lotusrainclinic.com/

Gary Foresman, MD
Middle Path Medicine
180 W. LePoint Street Unit A
Arroyo Grande, CA 93420
Phone: (805) 481-3442
Website: www.middlepathmedicine.com

Brent Hill, DC
Hill Center for Integrated Medicine
3609 Oakdale Rd., Suite 5
Modesto, CA 95357
Phone: (209) 551-8888
Website: www.hillwellness.com/

Paul Han Soo Kim, MD
Previ Medical Group
1776 Ygnacio Valley Rd., Suite 204
Walnut Creek, CA 94598
Phone: 925-691-7546
Website: www.previmedicalgroup.com/index.html

Leigh Erin Connealy, MD
Cancer Center for Healing
6 Hughes, Suite 120B
Irvine, CA 92618
Phone: 949-581-HOPE (4673)
E-mail: info@cancercenterforhealing.com
Website: www.cancercenterforhealing.com

Area of specialty: Targeted cancer therapies including IPTLD, high-dose vitamin C, hyperbaric oxygen therapy, ultraviolet blood irradiation, light beam generator, nutraceuticals, surgery, emotional therapies and more.

## COLORADO

Jonathan Singer, DO
8400 East Prentice Avenue, Suite 301
Greenwood Village, CO 80111
Phone: (303) 488-0034
Fax: (303) 488-0040
E-Mail: singerdo@aol.com
Website: www.denver-doctor.com

Johanne Wayne CN
Clinical Nutritionist
5762 W. Asbury Pl.
Lakewood, CO 80227
Tel: 303-916-5460
Fax: 303-484-6445
Email: johannewaynecn@live.com

Areas of specialty: Functional diagnostic nutrition & metabolic typing advisor level II

Brandon Lundell, DC Dipl Ac
619 Pratt St.
Longmont, CO 80501
Phone: (720) 771-0402
Fax: (303) 776-9272
E-mail: brandonlundell@juno.com

Roger Billica, MD
2362 East Prospect
Fort Collins, CO 80525
Phone: (970) 495-0999
Fax: (970) 495-1016
E-mail: trilifehealth@gmail.com or Website: www.trilifehealth.com/

## CONNETICUT

Stephen T. Sinatra, M.D., F.A.C.C.,
New England Heart Center
483 West Middle Tpke,
Manchester, CT 06040
Phone: (860) 643-5101
Fax: (860) 533-9747
Website: www.drsinatra.com

Dr. Nicholas J. Palermo, D.O.
257 East Center Street
Manchester, CT 06040
Phone: (860) 645-3927
Fax: (860) 643-2531
Email: DoctorPalermo@cox.net

Yvette Whitton, ND
Adonai Optimal Health and Wellness
31 Hawleyville Road
Newton, CT 06470
Phone: 888-655-8489

## DELAWARE

**Gertie Hillman, R.N.**
**Nutrition The Way To Life**
412 E. Savannah
Lewes, Delaware 11958
(302) 645-1696
Fax: (302) 645-4940

E-Mail: gerties.nutrition@verizon.net
(R.N. Hillman is a Certified Nutritionist and Herbalist and uses Poly-MVA in her Holistic Nutrition Counseling)

---

## FLORIDA

Jeffrey Mueller, MD
Whole Family Healthcare
1201 Louisiana Ave.
Ste. E
Winter Park, Florida 32792
Phone: (407) 644-2990
Fax: (407) 644-4370
Email: Reception@WholeFamilyHealthcare.com

Area of specialty: Whole Family Healthcare also features an unrivaled program for improving the quality of life in cancer patients and in those with virtually any chronic disease, with a special emphasis on improving nutrition and digestive issues.

This comprehensive, holistic clinic offers an intensive focus on lifestyle and dietary changes, Acupuncture, computerized health screenings, Chiropractic care, Qi Gong, massage therapy, Brain maps and Neurofeedback, a large natural pharmacy, and much more.
Martin Dayton, D.O., M.D.
Dayton Medica Ctr/Office
18600 Collins Avenue
Sunny Isles Beach, Florida 33160
Phone: (305) 931-8484
Email: drdayton@daytonmedical.com
Website: www.daytonmedical.com

John Monhollon, MD

Florida Integrative Medical Center
2415 University Parkway
Sarasota, FL 34243
Phone: (941) 955-6220
Website: www.floridaintegrative.com
Areas of specialty: Acupuncture, IV Therapy, Immune and Nutritional
Support, Holistic Dentistry and more.

Gene Wei, DOM, AP
Center for Acupuncture and Integrative Medicine
668 N. Orlando Avenue #1018
Maitland, FL 32751
Phone: (407) 622-8008
Website: www.caimedicine.com

Tammy Bennett, Doctor of Oriental Medicine
Susan Chapman, ARNP
Suma Wellness Centers
212 West Bay Avenue
Longwood, FL 34750
Phone: (407) 265-1888
Fax: (407) 265-9581
Email: tammy@longwoodhealingcenter.com
Website: www.sumawellness.com

Areas of specialty: Acupuncture, anti-aging medicine, functional medicine
and nutrition for cancer patients, bioidentical hormone therapy, holistic
pain management for cancer patients.

## GEORGIA
Nancy C. Farley, PhD
(Psychologist & Cancer Survivor)
625 Lexington Way
Woodstock, GA 30189

Phone: (770) 592-8775
E-mail: nfhaven@attbi.com

Veronique Desaulniers, DC
10863 Big Canoe
Jasper, GA 30143
Phone: (706) 579-2257
Website: www.breastcancerconqueror.com

## HAWAII
Ryan Ferchoff ND
The Natural Wellness Center
Naturopathic Physician
2752 Woodlawn Drive 5-110
Honolulu, HI 96822
Phone: (808)-988-0800
E-mail: INFO@TNWC.co
Website: www.thenaturalwellnesscenter.com

Areas of specialty: Wellness Retreat In-Patient Programs and Integrative Care, IV Therapies, Naturopathic Hospital, Cancer Support Programs and Treatments.

## IDAHO

Effie May Buckley, RN, MN
Choice Healing
18 Ponderosa Place
Boise, ID 83716
Phone: 208-429-8097
Website: www.choicehealing.net
Email: choicehealing@aol.com

Areas of specialty: Health Care, consultant, homeopathy, nutrition, neutriceuticals, energy medicine, diabetes, heavy metals.

## ILLINOIS

**Janet Fakhouri, N.D., N.C., M.S.**
**Custom Health, Inc.**
10748 South Cook Avenue
Oak Lawn, IL. 60453
708-261-7178

**James Corzine DC**
**Accident & Chronic Pain Center**
210 West Market Street
Christopher, Illinois 62822
Phone: 618-724-9200
E-mail: jcorzine@shawneelink.net

**Oscar I. Ordonez MD**
**Belvidere Center For Health & Nutrition**
6413 Logan Avenue, Suite 104
Belvidere, Illinois 61008
Phone: (815} 544-3112
Fax: {815) 544-3114
Email: OIOMD1@netzero.com

## INDIANA
Marvin Dziabis, M.D.
Health Restoration Clinic
107 W 7th St.

North Manchester, IN 46962
Phone: (260) 982-1400
Fax: (260) 982-1700
E-mail: dziabis@earthlink.net
Website: www.medical-library.net/doctors/health_restoration_clinic/

Dr. David J. Krizman
Center for Health Enrichment
322 N. Michigan St. Suite E
Plymouth, IN 46563
Phone: (574) 935-4000
Website: www.ptmc.azmyth.com

## IOWA
Frank Wiewel
People Against Cancer
604 East Street – P.O. Box 10
Otho, Iowa 50569 USA
Phone: 515-972-4444
Fax: 515-972-4415
E-Mail: info@PeopleAgainstCancer.net
Website: www.PeopleagainstCancer.net

## KANSAS

Bowers Natural Wellness
3450 N Rock Road Building 500 Suite 503
Wichita, KS 67226
Phone: (316) 636-5333
Fax: (316) 636-5338
E-mail: bnw@bnw.kscoxmail.com
Website: www.bowerswellness.com

Areas of specialty: Diplomate of the Chiropractic Board of Internal Diagnosis, Certified Functional Medicine Physician.

## MAINE

Sean McCloy, M.D., M.P.H.
Maine Integrative Wellness
222 Auburn St.
Portland, ME 04103
Phone: (207) 828-4299
Fax: (207) 828-5056

Email: drmccloy@mainewellness.com
Website: www.mainewellness.com

Fredric Shotz, N.D.
Maine Integrative Wellness
174 Falmouth Rd
Falmouth, Maine 04105
Phone: (207) 828-4299
Fax: (207) 828-5056

Email: drshotz@mainewellness.com
Website: www.mainewellness.com

## MARYLAND

Barbara Johnson, RN
3605 Southside Avenue
Phoenix, MD 21131-173
Phone: 410-628-6877
Email: bjohnsonrn@aol.com

Sholpan Yestekov, ND
Holistic Well-being
18514 Office Park Dr.
Gaithersburg, MD 20886
Phone: 301-366-1779
Email: sholpan@nes-kz.com
Website: www.holistic-wellbeing-health.com

Areas of specialty: Alternative and complementary medicine, Poly-MVA
and more to help support cancer patients.

## MICHIGAN

**Linda K. Hegstrand, MD, PhD**
**Blue Heron Academy of Healing Arts and Sciences**
2040 Raybrook SE Suite 104
Grand Rapids, MI 49546
Phone: 616-974-9004
E-Mail: Lhegstrand@aol.com

**Steven Margolis, M.D.**
**(Family Practice Physician)**
**Alternacare Clinic**
37300 Dequindre Road, Suite 201
Sterling Heights, Michigan 48310
Phone: 586-268-0228
Fax: 586-268-7392
E-Mail:Alternacare@hotmail.com

## MINNESOTA

Jean O'Hern, N.D.
Nature's Wisdom
2516 Lyndale Avenue South
Minneapolis, MN 55405
Phone: 612-872-4210
E-Mail: johern@usinternet.com

## MISSISSIPPI

**Dr. Arnold Smith, MD**
**North Central Mississippi Regional Cancer Center**
1401 River Road
Greenwood, MS 38930
Phone: 662-459-7133 Fax: 662-459-7136
Website: http://www.cancernet.com/

## MISSOURI

Wesley Delport, ND
Abundant Health and Wellness
4323 S. National Avenue
Springfield, MO 65810
Phone: (417) 890-7400
Toll Free: 800-528-7796
Email: abundanthealth@sbcglobal.net
Website: www.getwellnaturally.net

Stuart Hoover, NHD
Essential 2 Health

1358 E. Kingsley Street Suite C
Springfield, MO 65804
Phone: (417) 883-0115
Website: www.e2health.com

## NEVADA

James W. Forsythe, M.D., H.M.D.
Medical Oncologist and Homeopath
521 Hammill Lane
Reno, Nevada 89511
Phone: (775) 827-0707
Fax: (775) 827-1006
Website: www.drforsythe.com
Email: eforsythe@sbcglobal.net

Robert Eslinger, MD
Reno Integrative Medical Center
6110 Plumas Street, Suite B
Reno, NV 89519
Phone: (775) 829-1009

Website: www.renointegrativemedicalcenter.com

Terry Pfau, MD
Renaissance Health Center
2820 W. Charleston Blvd., Suite 6
Las Vegas, NV 89102
Phone: (702) 258-7860
Website: www.terrypfau-do.md.com/

## NEW JERSEY

Stuart H. Freedenfeld, MD
Stockton Family Practice
56 South Main St
Stockton, NJ 08559
Phone: 609-397-8585
E-mail: info@stocktonfp.com
Website: http://www.StocktonFP.com

Areas of Specialty: At Stockton Family Practice we have been offering cancer therapies for clients who wish complimentary support during chemotherapy or radiation treatments, for clients who have failed conventional therapies, and for those who choose not to pursue conventional chemotherapy.

We offer a wide range of services, from dietary interventions, nutritional supplements, and metabolic therapies, to acupuncture and intravenous therapies. We will develop an integrative program based on the specific needs and specific wishes of each individual.

Some of the therapies include enzymes, Antineoplastons, angiogenesis inhibitors, Vitamin C, Ozone, Poly-MVA, Haluronic acid, Ukraine and Amygdalin.

Molly Fantasia, PhD & Ronald Intelisano, DO
Associates In Preventive Medicine
1930 E. Marlton Pike, Suite J52
Cherry Hill, NJ 08003
Phone: 856-489-0505
Fax: 856-489-0435
E-mail: IVDOCS@aol.com
Website: www.cherryhillclinic.com

Areas of Specialty: Molly Fantasia, PhD – Fellow, American Association of Integrative Medicine. We provide therapy for: Auto-Immune Diseases, Cancer Support, Glutathione, Hydration Therapy, Preventative Medicine, Predictive Genomic Testing.

Allan Magaziner, DO
Magaziner Center for Wellness
1907 Greentree Road
Cherry Hill, NJ 08003
Phone: (856) 424-8222
Website: www.drmagaziner.com

## NEW YORK

Richard Linchitz, MD
Jesse A. Stoff, MD
Linchitz Medical Wellness
70 Glen Street, Suite 240
Glen Cove, NY 11542
516.759.4200
Website: http://www.linchitzwellness.com
Email: info@linchitzwellness.com

Moshe Dekel
166 Elaine Drive
Oceanside, NY 11572
Phone: 516-208-6617
Fax: 516-208-6617
E-mail: doc@drdekel.com
Website: www.drdekel.com

## NORTH CAROLINA

Rashid A. Buttar, DO, FACAM, FAAPM
Advanced Concepts In Alternative And Preventive Medicine
20721 Torrence Chapel Road, Suite 101 – 102
Cornelius, NC 28031
Phone: (704) 895-9355
Fax: (704) 895-9357
E-Mail: drbuttarclinic@aol.com
Website: www.drbuttar.com

Bill Crawford, M.D., Board Certified Naturopath
P.O. Box 995
Franklin, NC 28744
Phone: (828) 421-9336
Fax: (828) 349-1367

## OHIO

Marcus Cobb, MD
Healthy Pursuit Medical Center
7060 Ridgetop Drive
West Chester, OH 45069
Phone: (513) 779-4325
Fax: (513) 742-1296
E-Mail: marcuslcobb@mac.com

Theodore Togliatti MD
Steven Mann DO
Insook Chung RN MSN FNP
Get Well Center
635 S. Trimble Road
Mansfield, Ohio 44906

Phone: (419) 524-2676
Fax: (419) 524-2692
E-mail: ChungGWC@aol.com

Larry Everhart, MD
Host Nutrition
3779 Attucks Drive
Powell, OH 43065
Phone: (614) 718-9800

## OKLAHOMA

Mary Schrick, N.D.
Full Circle Health Clinic
3601 S. Broadway
Edmond, Oklahoma 73013
Phone: (405) 753-9355

Dr. Paul Rothwell, M.D.
Wellness and Longevity
7530 NW 23rd Street
Bethany, Oklahoma 73008
Phone: 405-787-8556
Fax: 405-787-7424
Email: info@wellnessok.com
Website: www.wellnessok.com

## TEXAS

Ashok Patel, MD
500 North Highway 67

Phone: (604) 273-4372
Website: www.drjimchan.com
E-Mail: info@drjimchan.com

## CYPRESS

Dr. George J Georgiou, Ph.D.,N.D.,DSc (AM).,MSc.,BSc
Holistic Medicine Practitioner DaVinci Natural Health Centre
Panayia Aimatousa 300, Aradippou 7101
Larnaca, Cyprus
Telephone: (+357) 24-82 33 22
Fax: (+357) 24- 82 33 21
E-Mail: admin@docgeorge.com
Website: www.docgeorge.com and www.collegenaturalmedicine.com

## DOMINICAN REPUBLIC

George Zabrecky, M.D.
The Americas Research & Treatment Center
El Vergel #45 Ortega y Gasset
Santa Domingo, Dominican Republic
Phone: (809) 472-1238
Fax: (809) 567-8386

## ITALY

Fiamma Ferraro, MD
Via Paganella 7A
00135 Roma,Italy
Phone: (+39)0635500018
Cell: (+39)3403754383
E-Mail: fer@yahoo.com
Website: www.geocities.com/fiafer

**JAPAN**
Andrew Wong, MD, PhD
Roppongi Dr. Andy`s Clinic of Plastic & Cosmetic
Surgery and Age Management Medicine
6/7 F Roppongi Shimada Bldg.,
4-8-7, Roppongi, Minato-ku
Tokyo, Japan 106-0032
Phone: 81-3-3401-0720
Fax: 81-3-3401-0704
E-mail: andy@drandy.com
Web Page: www.drandy.com

**LEBANON**
Tony Georges Lichaa, M.D.
(Specialist in Internal Medicine & Cardiology Trained at the Montreal
Heart Institute, American Board of Chelation Therapy)

Beirut Location:

The Anti-Aging and Life Rejuvenating
Medical Center
Verdun Plaza One, 2nd Floor
Beirut, Lebanon
Phone: 961 3 25 49 45
Email: tlichaa@inco.com.lb

Jounieh Location:

The Medical Center For Prevention And The Treatment Of Diseases
P.O. Box 245
Jounieh, Lebanon

Phone: 961 9 911 875
Fax: 961 9 914 195
Email: tlichaa@inco.com.lb

## MANITOBA

Dr. Jim Chan, N.D.
EuroMed Foundation
3331-No. 3 Road
Richmond, BC V6X 2B6
Phone: (604) 273-4372
Email: info@drjimchan.com
Website: www.drjimchan.com

Dennis Wong, B.Sc. Pharm., FAARFM, CCN, ABAAHP
CD Whyte Ridge Pharmacy Specialty Compounding & Integrative
Consultation services
123 Scurfield Blvd.
Winnipeg, MB
Phone: 204-488-1819
Fax: 204-489-2828

CinDen Pharmacy
1600 Pembina Hwy.
Winnipeg, MB R3T 5Z2
Phone: 204-452-7989
Fax 204-452-7585
Email: dennis@cdwhyteridgerx.com
Website: www.cdwhyteridgerx.com

Area of specialty: Clinical Consultant Pharmacist /owner; Fellow, Anti-Aging, Regenerative & Functional Medicine; Certified Clinical Nutritionist; Diplomat, American Board of Anti-Aging Health Practitioners.

**MEXICO**
Playas de Tijuana, B.C.
Phone: 1-855-366-4673
Fax: 1-619-956-7071
Website: www.h4cmedical.com
E-mail: Info@h4cmedical.com

Recommended Therapies Could Include: Sono-Photo Dynamic Therapy, Poly MVA, Insulin Potentiation Therapy, Hyperthermia, Enzyme Therapy, IV Therapy, Iscador, Laetrile, Detoxification, and Anti-Cancer Vaccines. The anti-cancer programs at Hope4Cancer Institute are specifically designed to meet the needs of each individual patients.

Jorge Llamas, MD
Paseo Playas #400 Secc. Terrazas
Playas de Tijuana, B.C.
Mexico Phone: 664-680-1484
U.S. Phone: 619-752-9903
Cell Phone: 664-188-5533
E-mail: Dr_llamas@hotmail.com
Metabolic Therapies: Hyperthermia (Whole Body) and Local Indiba, I.P.T., Galuanotherapy, Oxygen Therapy, Homo-Acupuncture, Nutrition

Exiquio Cardenas, Medico Alapata/Naturopata
Piedras Negras, Coahuila
E-mail: Dr.naturista@hotmail.com
Areas of Specialty: Mas de 30 anos de experiencia en terapias alternativas no farmacologicas, terapia de Bowen, biomagnetismo, auriculoterapia, herbolaria Ayurvedica, reiki, healing touch, terapia celular, Master Tung's acupuncture, nutricion naturista, medicina antienvejecimiento, deintoxicacion intensiva, etc.

There is a bright future for patients who make choices for bettering their health and gaining complete healing through natural and alternative therapies.

**If you wish to have 6 months free of updates on breast cancer. Send an e-mail to cancergroup@gmail.com along with your order number.**

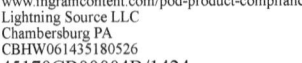